CANCER
AND
VITAMIN C

CANCER
AND
VITAMIN C

A DISCUSSION OF THE NATURE, CAUSES, PREVENTION,
AND TREATMENT OF CANCER WITH SPECIAL REFERENCE
TO THE VALUE OF VITAMIN C

Ewan Cameron, M.B., Ch.B., F. R. C. S. (Glasgow), F. R. C. S. (Edinburgh)

and

Linus Pauling, Ph.D.

WARNER BOOKS

A Warner Communications Company

A Warner Communications Company

Printed in the United States of America

First printing: June 1981

10 9 8 7 6 5 4 3 2 1

Cover design by New Studio

Library of Congress Cataloging in Publication Data

Cameron. Ewan.
  Cancer and vitamin C.

  Reprint of the 1979 ed. published by Linus Pauling
Institute of Science and Medicine. Menlo Park. Calif.
  Bibliography: p.
  Includes indexes.
  1. Vitamin C—Therapeutic use. 2. Cancer—
Chemotherapy. 3. Cancer. I. Pauling. Linus. 1901–
joint author. II. Title. [DNLM: 1. Neoplasms.
2. Neoplasms—Drug therapy. 3. Ascorbic acid—
Therapeutic use. QZ267 C182c 1979a]
[RC271.A78C35 1981]   616.99'4061   80-21382
ISBN 0-446-97735-7 (U.S.A.)
ISBN 0-446-97852-3 (Canada)

Contents

Preface   ix

Part I.   THE NATURE AND CAUSES OF CANCER   1

CHAPTER 1   The Nature of Cancer   3
        2   The Causes of Cancer   10
        3   The Common Forms of Human Cancer   18

Part II.   THE TREATMENT OF CANCER   45

        4   The Treatment of Cancer   47
        5   The Treatment of Cancer by Surgery   50
        6   The Treatment of Cancer by Radiotherapy   58
        7   The Treatment of Cancer by Chemotherapy   62
        8   The Treatment of Cancer by Hormones   70
        9   The Treatment of Cancer by Immunotherapy   78
       10   Some Unconventional Forms of Cancer Treatment   83

Part III.   A RATIONAL APPROACH TO THE TREATMENT
            OF CANCER   87

       11   Controlling Cancer   89
       12   Spontaneous Regressions in Cancer   93
       13   Host Resistance to Cancer   96
       14   Vitamin C   99
       15   Vitamin C and the Immune System   108
       16   Other Properties of Vitamin C   112
       17   The Utilization of Vitamin C by Cancer Patients   120

Part IV.   THE USE OF VITAMIN C IN THE TREATMENT
           AND PREVENTION OF CANCER   127

      18   The Principal Trial of Vitamin C
           in Vale of Leven Hospital   129
      19   Other Clinical Trials   140
      20   Case Histories of Vale of Leven Patients   146
      21   Some Illustrative Patients from the
           United States and Canada   168
      22   The Prevention of Cancer   183
      23   Summary and Conclusions: The Role of
           Vitamin C in the Treatment of Cancer   189

APPENDIX I   Estimated Cancer Deaths in the
              United States for 1980   197
       II   Foods and Nutrition   199
      III   Some Information about Anticancer Drugs   203
       IV   Practical Information about Vitamin C and its Use   208
        V   A Discussion of Surgical Terms   211

            Glossary   217
            References   223
            Name Index   229
            Subject Index   231

Preface

Some years ago we developed the idea that regular high intakes of vitamin C (ascorbic acid, or its several biologically active salts known as ascorbates) play some part both in the prevention of cancer and in the treatment of established cancer.

Evidence steadily accumulates to support this view.

Cancer, of course, is the major unsolved health problem with strong emotional overtones. Although not the major killer, it has become the most feared of all diseases and a major focus of biological research throughout the world. The repeated statement of our views and clinical results in the scientific literature has given rise to much fruitful discussion with colleagues in the scientific and medical fields, and it has also involved us in a massive correspondence with desperate cancer patients seeking advice and help, as well as with their families, friends, and physicians.

For some years we have tried to write personal letters to these patients, family members, friends, and physicians, but meeting this obligation is now beyond our resources. It seems increasingly clear to us that many of these despairing patients lack understanding of (a) the very nature of cancer, (b) the value and the limitations of all conventional (and some unconventional) forms of treatment of cancer, and (c) our own views as to how vitamin C might help them. This book is an attempt to answer these questions.

Cancer is an unpleasant disease. Death by cancer usually involves much more suffering than other ways of death, such as by a heart attack. The cancer patient may lead a life of misery for months or years before his suffering is brought to an end by death. Much of his misery may be caused by the treatment that is given him in the effort to control the disease.

In the United States about 1.9 million people will die this year. About 20 percent of the deaths, 395,000, will be from cancer. Every day about 2,100 people in this country develop cancer and about 1,080 die of cancer. If the incidence and mortality continue at their present rates, one adult in the United States in every three will develop cancer at some time in his life, and one in five will die of the disease.

During the last twenty years about ten billion dollars has been spent on cancer research, in the effort to get some control of the disease. The budget of the National Cancer Institute for the year 1979 is $900 million and that of the American Cancer Society is $140 million. Despite this great expenditure and the corresponding great effort, not much has been achieved. Some progress has been made in the treatment of some kinds of cancer, especially leukemia and Hodgkin's disease, by new regimes of treatment with high-energy radiation and anticancer drugs. For most kinds of cancer, those involving solid tumors in adults, which lead to 95 percent of the cancer deaths, there has been essentially no change in overall incidence and mortality during recent years.

One of us (Ewan Cameron) is a surgeon who for over thirty years has been involved in the treatment of cancer patients. During the early part of this period he developed the idea that the most important factor determining the progress and outcome of any cancer illness is the natural resistance of the patient to his disease. In his 1966 book *Hyaluronidase and Cancer* he pointed out that the resistance of the normal tissues surrounding a malignant tumor to infiltration by that tumor would be increased if the strength of the intercellular cement (also called ground substance) that binds the cells of the normal tissues together could be increased. This intercellular cement contains very long molecular chains, called glycosaminoglycans, that give it strength, and it also contains fibrils of the protein collagen, which further strengthen the cement in the same way as the steel reinforcing rods strengthen reinforced concrete. It is in fact known that some, and probably all, malignant tumors liberate an enzyme, hyaluronidase, that causes the glycosaminoglycans to be cut into smaller molecules, thus weakening the intercellular cement. Moreover, some, and perhaps all, malignant tumors also liberate another enzyme, collagenase, that causes the collagen fibrils to be split into small molecules, further weakening the normal tissues and making it easier for the malignant tumor to grow into them in the way characteristic of malignancies.

These facts indicate clearly that the effort should be made to strengthen the intercellular cement in the normal tissues of cancer patients and to inhibit the tumor enzymes that cause its breakdown. Until 1971, however, no one had found a way of doing this. Then in that year two new ideas, both involving vitamin C, were advanced. Cameron and Douglas Rotman, on the basis of some chemical arguments, suggested that an increased concentration of vitamin C in the body would stimulate the normal cells to produce increased amounts of the substance hyaluronidase inhibitor, which would combine with the enzyme hyaluronidase liberated by the malignant tumor and prevent it from attacking the intercellular cement. At the same time the other author of this book (Linus Pauling) pointed out that it is known that vitamin C is required for the synthesis of collagen; accordingly increasing the intake of this vitamin would cause more collagen fibrils to be made, further strengthening the intercellular cement.

He suggested to Cameron, for reasons discussed in Chapter 14, that an intake of 10 grams of vitamin C per day be given to the patients with advanced cancer. Clinical trials were cautiously begun by Cameron in Vale of Leven Hospital, Loch Lomondside, Scotland, in November 1971. The patients who were treated with vitamin C during the first year were those with advanced cancer for whom the conventional treatments had ceased to be of benefit —patients considered in Scottish medical practice to be "untreatable."

Cameron soon was convinced that most of the patients who received vitamin C benefited from it, and with each succeeding year a larger fraction of the cancer patients in this hospital were given the vitamin. Over 500 patients in this hospital with advanced cancer and many with cancer in earlier stages have received vitamin C, in conjunction with other therapy, during the eight years since this treatment was instituted. The use of vitamin C has also spread to other hospitals in this region of Scotland, and to a smaller extent to other parts of the world.

The first observation that was made is that for many cancer patients the administration of vitamin C seems to improve the state of well-being, as measured by improved appetite, increased mental alertness, decreased requirement for pain-killing drugs, and other clinical criteria. This effect was described by Cameron and Campbell (1974) in their report on the first 50 ascorbate-treated patients in the following words:

> We should now like to describe what we have come to recognize as the standard response to large-dose ascorbic acid supplements in patients with advanced cancer. Subjective evidence of benefit is usually apparent by about the 5th to 10th day of treatment, and in many patients this response can be very striking indeed. The patient then enters a stage of increased well-being and general clinical improvement, and during this phase objective evidence accumulates to confirm that some retardation of tumor growth has been achieved. The objective evidence of benefit varies with the individual clinical presentation, but may take the form of relief of particularly distressing pressure symptoms such as pain from skeletal metastases, a slowing down of the rate of accumulation of malignant effusions, a trend toward improvement in malignant jaundice, or relief from respiratory distress, and is accompanied by a slow fall in the erythrocyte sedimentation rate and the serum seromucoid concentration. This phase of clinical improvement may be

very transient, or it may last for weeks or months, and in a few patients may be so prolonged and accompanied by such convincing evidence of objective benefit as to indicate that permanent regression has been induced.

An unexpected and potentially valuable relation of vitamin C to addictive narcotic drugs was also noted. Many patients with advanced cancer, especially those with skeletal metastases, suffer severe pain because of the pressure developed by the growth of the tumor in a restricted space. This pain frequently requires the use of narcotic drugs. Cameron and Baird (1973) reported that the first five ascorbate-treated patients who had been receiving large doses of morphine or heroin to control pain were taken off these drugs a few days after the treatment with vitamin C was begun, because the vitamin C seemed to diminish the pain to such an extent that the drug was not needed. Moreover, none of these patients asked that the morphine or heroin be given to them —they seemed not to experience any serious withdrawal signs or symptoms. This observation was the basis of the recently reported successful use of massive doses of vitamin C in the treatment of narcotic addiction (Libby and Stone, 1976).

A careful study has been made of 100 of the first ascorbate-treated cancer patients in Vale of Leven Hospital, in comparison with 1000 cancer patients who were matched (10 to 1) with the ascorbate-treated patients with respect to age, sex, type of cancer, and clinical state and who were treated by the same physicians, in the same hospital, and in the same way except that they did not receive the doses of vitamin C. The results of this study were reported in two papers (Cameron and Pauling, 1976, 1978) and are discussed in detail in later chapters of this book, beginning with Chapter 18. Here we may mention that on the average the ascorbate-treated patients survived ten months longer than their matched controls. Twenty-two of the 100 ascorbate-treated patients (22 percent) lived longer than a year after being deemed to have reached the terminal stage, whereas only four of the 1000 controls (0.4 percent) lived this long. The average survival time of these 22 ascorbate-treated patients after being deemed terminal has now (15 September 1979) reached 2.8 years, and continues to increase with the passing of time because five of these patients are still alive; all of the controls have died.

In this study, in which the treatment with vitamin C was introduced only in the terminal phase of the illness, most of the patients were not so fortunate. After a period of sustained clinical improvement the malignant activity reasserted itself, and the patient died from his original disease. In many of these patients the mode of death was in itself unusual. After a period of comparative well-being and apparent tumor quiescence the patient very suddenly entered a rapid terminal phase with a precipitous downhill course and death within a few days from fulminating cancer. In some patients these events followed immediately the cessation, for one reason or another, of the intake of the large doses of vitamin C, and for these patients the rapid decline may well be attributed to this action. For other patients, however, who continued to receive the vitamin some other explanation of the sudden transition from apparent restraint to uncontrolled dissemination of the malignancy is needed. There is still uncertainty about the most effective dosage of vitamin C for cancer patients, and it is possible that permanent regression could have been achieved for some of these patients by giving them larger doses of the vitamin. In fact, amounts larger than 10 grams per day—as much as 100 grams per day—have been used in some cancer patients, both by intravenous infusion and orally, with apparent benefit. In one patient recurrence of the cancer that had been controlled for six months by intake of 10 grams per day was observed to follow the cessation of intake of the vitamin. The recurrent cancer did not respond to oral doses of 10 grams per day for 10 days but did respond by a second regression to 20 grams by intravenous infusion for 10 days, followed by a maintenance oral dosage of 12½ grams per day (Cameron, Campbell, and Jack, 1975; see also Chapter 20).

Many patients with cancer in earlier stages in Vale of Leven Hospital and elsewhere have been treated with a large intake of vitamin C, in conjunction with other therapeutic measures, often with great apparent benefit. No carefully controlled long-term trial to determine the amount of this benefit has been carried out. We believe, however, on the basis of our own observations (some of which are discussed in later chapters of this book) that vitamin C therapy against cancer is much more effective when it is begun early in the development of the disease than when it is postponed until the patient has reached the apparently hopeless stage.

There is also much evidence that an increased intake of vitamin C by healthy people significantly decreases the chance of developing cancer. This evidence is discussed in Chapter 22.

We have some information about how vitamin C works in the prevention and treatment of cancer, but much remains to be discovered. Vitamin C can inactivate viruses by a molecular mechanism that is understood, and it may function in this way to help control those human cancers that are thought to involve viruses. It also has rather general detoxifying powers for toxic substances that enter the human body, including carcinogenic chemicals (substances that cause cancer). Probably its most important modes of action are those in which it increases the effectiveness of the body's natural protective mechanisms, especially the various immune mechanisms. A detailed discussion of the mechanisms of action of vitamin C is given in Chapters 15 and 16.

It is our opinion that supplemental vitamin C has value for the prevention of all forms of cancer in healthy human beings and also is of some benefit in the treatment of patients with cancer in every stage of the disease, and can be of great value to some patients. We believe that before long the use of this simple, safe, natural, and inexpensive substance will become an accepted part of all regimes for the prevention and treatment of cancer.

Our work has been supported in part by The Educational Foundation of America, the Foundation for Nutritional Advancement, the Pioneer Fund, and the Linus Pauling Institute of Science and Medicine. For their help in various ways, we thank Dr. Allan Campbell, Dr. J. Ross Maccallum, Dr. James Enstrom, Dr. Linus Pauling, Jr., Professor Crellin Pauling, Helen C. Nauts, Brian Leibovitz, Morton Klein, Anita Maclaren, and Margaret Sheen. We are grateful also to W. H. Freeman and Company and its staff for their assistance in producing the book, and the members of the staff of the Linus Pauling Institute, who have contributed to the writing of this book in many ways.

Ewan Cameron
Linus Pauling

Linus Pauling Institute of Science and Medicine
2700 Sand Hill Road, Menlo Park, California 94025

CANCER
AND
VITAMIN C

PART I
THE NATURE AND CAUSES OF CANCER

1

The Nature
of Cancer

The human body may be compared with a clay sculpture. Corresponding to the internal wire frame of the sculpture, we have a bony skeleton, which is hinged here and there to permit motion. In order to give this structure life and being there are some 10 trillion (10,000,000,000,000) cells scattered throughout, occupying, together with the body fluids, every available interstice. Each cell carries out some specialized functions. They range from those of the simple fibroblast, which is busily at work keeping the reinforcing material in good shape, and the lymphocytes and other white cells, which destroy invading bacteria and cancer cells, to the highly complex cells of the brain, which formulate and transmit the orders for all this corporate activity and which interact with one another in such a way as to fashion our consciousness, provide our memory bank, and permit us to think and reason. To hold the cells together and to fill us out to shapely proportions we have a ubiquitous material called the *ground substance* or intercellular cement, mentioned in the preface. Thoroughly mixed into this ground substance is a dense network of collagen and other fibers to give it extra strength and resilience.

These 10 trillion cells all function as subservient members of one highly integrated unit, the human body, obedient to the motto "Each for all, and all for one." They can be likened to the members of a highly organized national state with an extremely strict code of law and order, with each individual performing his allotted task for the good of the whole and with any disobedience or failure to serve the collective organization punished by immediate expulsion and death.

Most of these cells have the capacity for infinite multiplication and also for reversion to a more primitive and less specialized form. This capacity is demonstrated in the technique of tissue culture: a normal cell is taken from a human being or other organism and put in a glass flask where it is provided with the right nutrients and kept at the right temperature; it then divides into two cells, and the process of cell division continues without end, producing a vast succession of generations of progeny, so long as we provide the requisite artificial environment.

This capacity for repeated multiplication is continually operating in the perfectly healthy body, but always in a very carefully controlled manner. Cells of some kinds in the human body age and die and are constantly being replaced by fresh offspring, but always within the total ceiling of 10 trillion. Skin is a good example. Our complexion consists of a smooth patina of dead cells that are constantly being discarded and just as constantly being replaced by generations of new cells rising up from the deeper living layer, and yet the whole process is so nicely regulated and controlled throughout our whole lifespan that only a very few unfortunate persons, with rare genetic diseases, ever develop rhinoceros hides or pathologically thin skins because of a fault in this regulatory mechanism. The specialized cells of the gastrointestinal tract, millions and millions of them arranged in fronds and villi to increase their functional area and busily secreting digestive enzymes and absorbing the processed nutrients for distribution to their compatriots, also wear out and die and are then discarded, broken down into small molecules for recycling or elimination, to be automatically replaced by fresh vigorous young descendants ready to carry on the same function—and yet for most human beings we do not see an intestine choked and blocked by solid masses of such cells or a useless intestine completely devoid of them.

The proliferative capacity of cells is best seen in the process of repair after injury. In any healthy tissue of an adult at any time we have a stable number of cells that divide only now and then to replace their defunct brethren. But when a wound is inflicted on that tissue everything is galvanized into frenzied activity. All cells in the immediate vicinity leap into action, dividing rapidly to repair the defect. It is interesting to note that if one takes a small sample of such healing tissue and submits it to an experienced histopathologist without telling him that it has come from a recent wound his opinion after microscopic examination of the tissue may be that it is from a malignant tumor. But of course it is not malignant, because as soon as the healing process is complete the cells revert to their usual well-controlled existence and their life continues as before the injury.

This almost unbelievably precise and quite magnificent control mechanism enables the human being to survive as a completely integrated functioning organism, instead of turning into a heterogeneous mass of warring cellular factions.

Cancer occurs when a cell and its descendants (or sometimes two or more cells of different kinds and their descendants) escape from this control mechanism and begin to behave in a renegade fashion. When we consider the total number of cells at risk and their continuing activity throughout life, we must conclude that the remarkable fact is not that people develop cancer, but rather that many people escape this fate throughout their lives.

Thus cancer occurs when a single cell (or a group of a few cells) escapes from regulatory control and is able to bequeath its independence to its descendants through every succeeding generation. The cancer cell exploits his new-found freedom to the utmost. No longer need he stay in place, wait in line for food, nor perform any function for the benefit of the whole organism. He can reproduce at will, building up an immense clone of equally ruthless offspring. Suddenly he and his offspring can travel throughout the body, taking over new areas of territory and, by leaping in and out of the circulatory systems, establish new colonies of equally ruthless aggressors in distant lands. He has acquired the trick of securing the lion's share of the available nutrients. He may cease to perform the functions that he formerly carried out for the benefit of the whole community of cells. He is the true wayward renegade rebel, creating his own largely independent colony within the corporate state of the human body.

For a time he may enjoy great success. He is efficient and aggressive. He and his progeny have the potential to be truly immortal, except for one thing: they are parasites who need the food, water, and oxygen and all sorts of metabolic services provided by the rest of the organism. The cancer cell attacks, has his initial success, enjoys a brief moment of supremacy, and then, as the source of the essential supporting services is destroyed, he also dies.

In the following paragraphs we outline the progressive stages of development, establishment, and dissemination of human cancer.

Although undoubtedly many changes go before, the first clearly detectable stage is that of *precancer*. Evidence of this stage may be seen by use of the optical microscope, which reveals changes in the appearance and configuration of cells that predict frank malignant change. In healthy epithelium (outer layer) of the skin, for example, the microscopist has before him an orderly array of identically shaped cells, each with its own sharply defined nucleus and each neatly mortised into its neighbors in a nearly perfect pattern of uniform thickness. But in precancerous change there is an obvious irregularity of the epithelial thickness, with peaks and troughs related to the profusion or scarcity of the component cells. Furthermore, the cells have lost their uniformity; there are dwarf cells and giant cells interspersed with cells of normal size, and many cells show gross irregularity of the nuclei. This development of structural irregularity and confusion often precedes clinical cancer, but not always, as will be discussed in later chapters.

We may assume that such precancerous changes occur in every tissue, although their identification is possible only in situations accessible for surveillance. These are in the epithelium of the cervix of the uterus (by the Pap-smear technique), in the breast (by biopsy for intra-duct carcinoma), and in the urinary bladder (search for the so-called unstable transitional uroepithelium). What are observed are visibly abnormal cells, proliferating in an irregular fashion and clearly associated with malignant change, but as yet showing no migration and no evidence of malignant invasiveness.

The next stage is frank local cancer. Here the distortion of individual cell structure is more pronounced, with a tendency to reversion to a more primitive "undifferentiated" type of cells, and, more important, with infiltration of the abnormal cells from their normal locations into the surrounding tissues.

There are several grades at this stage, building up to the sizeable local "lump" or tumor that needs no microscope for its recognition. The tumor (which is called the *primary tumor*) consists of a steadily expanding mass of subdividing cells. It can grow rapidly: in only 25 cell divisions (25 generations) a single cancerous cell can have over 30 million progeny, forming a tumor the size of a baseball, if no loss of tumor cells takes place.

At this time signs and symptoms usually become evident. The mass, lump, tumor, or cancer (meaning the same, if it is a malignant growth) may have reached such size as to be recognized. If it is of the skin, we may see it as an indolent (painless) ulcer that will not heal; if it is in a prominent structure, such as the breast, we can begin to feel it as a suspiciously hard nodule different in consistency from the normal tissues. Elsewhere it might make its intrinsically painless progress known indirectly by the slow compression of involved or adjacent structures, producing such effects as increasing difficulty in swallowing in cancer of the esophagus, obstruction of the large bowel and consequent problems of elimination in cancer of the colon, difficulty in urination in cancer of the prostate, painless jaundice because of compression of the bile duct by cancer of the pancreas, and hoarseness caused by compression of the nerve to the larynx by hilar cancer of the bronchus (lung cancer). Or it might declare its presence by suddenly ulcerating through some vital membrane, producing anything from barely noticeable to massive bleeding, such as hemoptysis (coughing up blood), hematemesis (vomiting blood), melena (passing blood in the stools), vaginal bleeding (from some ulcerative lesion in the female generative tract), or hematuria (passing blood in the urine). Every one of these signs and symptoms can be caused by disorders other than cancer and the probability of some other cause is greater than that of cancer, but every such manifestation of disease must be thoroughly checked out. Whether the clinical presentation is dramatic or trivial, we may at this stage be dealing with early local cancer, with significant possibility of successful treatment.

If we look at such an established tumor through a microscope we see a mob of cancer cells producing their progeny—in technical terms,"undifferentiated cells showing a high mitotic rate." Depending upon the growth rate of the particular tumor (to be discussed in later chapters), these cells bear less and less resemblance to their original progenitor. In tumors of relatively slow growth the malignant cells, although abnormal, still bear the clear imprint of their tissue and particular cell type of origin in their general appearance, behavior, and relative spatial configuration. In contrast, the cells in fast-growing tumors are so primitive and undifferentiated ("anaplastic") that they could have arisen from almost any tissue.

The expanding mass of new cells ("neoplasia") will first stretch and distend the neighboring structures as it grows, demonstrating one of the two main features of neoplastic cell behavior, *uncontrolled proliferation.* Very soon the other main feature, *invasiveness,* becomes apparent. Cells at the periphery of the tumor are driven outwards to infiltrate the surrounding tissue, spreading along the paths of least resistance between the layers of the tissues and being deflected by barriers such as epithelial layers, muscle sheaths, tendons, cartilage, and bone. It soon becomes obvious, however, that this infiltration is an active process, and that the infiltrating cells have the ability to digest away almost any barrier in their path. Soon we have a central tumor with spreading tentacles radiating outwards, destroying everything in their way, a true "Cancer" (the Latin word for crab). If such a tumor is close to a surface—the skin or the lining of the stomach, intestine, bladder, or bronchus—it will destroy the lining to form an enlarging malignant ulcer. The tumor will grow, spread, and destroy, but so long as it is confined to its parent organ it is called a Stage-I cancer.

The next step is usually the spread to the *lymph glands* (lymph nodes) in the region of the primary tumor. Most tissues are permeated by innumerable lymphatics. These lymphatics are fine thin-walled vessels that drain tissue fluid to filter stations, the regional lymph nodes. Familiar examples are the glands of the groin that drain the legs and those of the armpits that drain the arms and the breast. The regional lymph nodes in turn pass their lymph on to the next group of glands in the system. Thus the glands of the groin drain to glands deep in the pelvis, which in turn drain upwards through glands grouped around the aorta and others in the back of the chest, and the ramifications of the whole system come together at one point on the left side of the neck, where the body-wide lymph enters the venous system. The lymphatic system plays an important part in protecting the body against many diseases, including cancer.

The erosive ability of the tumor cells soon opens a way into the lymphatic system. Clumps of tumor cells enter the breached lymphatic, and either are carried along by the rather sluggish flow of the lymph or, more commonly, grow along the lymphatic to reach the first lymph node, where they are stopped by its filtering action. Perhaps at this stage many of these invaders are destroyed by the lymphocytes in the lymph node, but the usual progression is that they succeed in establishing a foothold, flourish, and eventually destroy the lymph node. The process then continues to the next node in the chain. An invaded lymph node steadily increases in size, and if accessible becomes easily felt. Sometimes enlargement of a lymph node is the first sign of the disease. It is not uncommon for a woman to discover an invaded node in her armpit when neither she nor her physician can palpate the small primary tumor in her breast. There is some confusion about nomenclature, but most surgeons would assign the designation Stage-II cancer to a tumor still apparently confined to its organ of origin except for the involvement of the regional lymph nodes draining that organ.

Meanwhile the untreated tumor is still growing, invading outward from its primary location. The tumor may then infiltrate some adjacent organ or structure. Thus a cancer of the gallbladder may directly invade the adjacent liver or a cancer of the stomach may invade the adjacent pancreas or colon. Whether or not this is happening, the lymphatic spread may by this time have extended well beyond the regional lymph nodes, as when a cancer of the breast that has involved the armpit lymph nodes then appears in the nodes in the neck. Such advancement of the disease indicates a poorer prognosis, and most surgeons would categorize this situation as a Stage-III cancer.

The final stage, Stage IV, is dissemination by the blood stream to distant sites. Blood vessels, having thicker walls, are more resistant to invasion than lymphatics, but eventually they too succumb. Clumps of tumor cells enter the blood stream and are swiftly borne to where fortune takes them, which can be almost anywhere in the body. They move along the large blood vessels without hindrance, taking this branch or that until they lodge in a vessel too narrow to let them pass. There they erode their way out of the blood vessel and set up a new thriving colony. This colony is called a *metastasis* or a *secondary tumor*. These metastases are identical in appearance and behavior to the primary tumor, being simply progeny establishing themselves at distant sites. The metastases also grow, invade, destroy, spread, and metastasize. Stage-IV cancer has a very grave prognosis. It represents the moment of supreme but short-lived triumph for the cancer-cell rebellion. Soon some vital structure will break down, and the patient will die, and all the parasitic cancer cells will die with him.

The gloomy picture that we have just described is, of course, that of untreated cancer in a person whose natural powers of resistance are not strong enough to overcome the enemy. Even without treatment the picture is not always so gloomy. It is likely that cancer cells develop in every person, perhaps even several times in his life, that are recognized as abnormal by his inborn system of molecular surveillance and are then destroyed by his army of scavenger cells. Even a far advanced cancer sometimes disappears, to the happiness of the patient and his family and the surprise and puzzlement of the physician. These cases of so-called "spontaneous regression" are rare, but there is no doubt that they do occur. Also, it is almost certain that they occur because something has stimulated and potentiated the body's natural protective mechanisms to such an extent that they finally succeed in overcoming the enemy. Some tumors never develop effective metastases, and, moreover, some tumors grow so slowly as to make little or no difference to the patient's life and well-being. Moreover, surgery and other therapeutic regimes, such as use of high-energy radiation, chemotherapy, hormones, and immunostimulants, are sometimes successful in reversing or significantly slowing down the course of the disease. But, unfortunately, the worst cancer situation that we have described above occurs all too often—in fact, in about half of the persons who are recognized as having developed the disease. In later chapters of this book we discuss the steps that we believe can be taken to improve this situation.

2

The Causes
of Cancer

At this moment more than one million Americans are under medical care for cancer. This year about 395,000 of them will die, one every minute and a half (see Appendix I). And, of course, we must not think only of the United States. This is a world problem, and from that wider perspective we see that every four seconds a human being, with all his hopes and aspirations, is dying from cancer, possibly quite miserably.

These statistics are frightening.

What is the cause of all this suffering?

In a more innocent age, cancer was regarded as an act of God. We are now beginning to realize that many, and indeed probably the majority, of human cancers are man-made, the results of our careless and almost criminal pollution of our environment.

The first recognition of an environmental cause of cancer is attributed to Sir Percival Pott, a London surgeon who in 1775 described the cancer of the scrotum that was prevalent among the adolescent chimney sweeps of his day as an occupational disease. Since their early childhood they had been, to quote Sir Percival, "thrust up narrow and sometimes hot chimneys." His conclusion was that "the disease in these people seems to derive its origin from the lodgement of soot in the rugae (skin creases) of the scrotum." Thus over two centuries ago there was given a clear and concise description of a "cause-and-effect" occupational cancer, and more than an inkling as to how it might be prevented. Early in the present century patient work in a Japanese laboratory (the daily painting of a rabbit's ears with soot suspensions for week after week) did prove that soot (and later some of its identifiable chemical constituents) is indeed *carcinogenic*—able to give rise to cancer.

In later years many other forms of occupational cancer were recognized. When the causative carcinogen was identified it became possible to institute and enforce preventive measures and thus to eliminate the hazard. One of these diseases was the "Mule-spinners cancer" of the "Dark Satanic Cotton Mills" of Victorian England, again a scrotal cancer, caused by the constant saturation of work clothes by hot lubricating oil splashing from the steam-powered looms. Then there was the recognition of an abnormally high incidence of lung cancer among the uranium miners of Joachimsthal in Bohemia, where only much later was it recognized that the ores are highly radioactive and that the radioactive gas radon is present in the air. The solid radioactive decay products of the inhaled radon were deposited in the lungs, where they produced carcinogenic rays. About one half of the miners who had died up to 1939 had developed lung cancer. There was also the belated recognition in Germany and Russia, and later in the United States and Britain, of an abnormally high incidence of bladder cancer among workers in the aniline dyestuffs industry and other industries who were exposed to the substance β-naphthylamine. More recently it has been recognized that workers and other people exposed to asbestos have a high incidence of an unusually vicious cancer of the pleura and peritoneum, and even more alarmingly that this increased incidence occurs in family members whose only contact with asbestos came through the dust brought home on the workers' clothes. There was a particularly high incidence of this rather rare form of cancer in Japan that has been explained by the fact that the rice that they ate had been polished with asbestos fibers. An increased incidence of cancer has been observed also in other industries and many carcinogenic agents have been identified, such as carbon black in print workers, carbon tetrachloride in dry cleaners, benz-pyrene in roofing, asphalt, and coke oven workers, polychlorobiphenyls in paper-mill workers, vinyl chloride in the plastics industry, and many more.

Then came the clear demonstration of the link between cigarette smoking and lung cancer. Cigarette smoking became fashionable among men in the 1920s, and about 25 years later the world experienced an explosive growth of lung cancer among men. Between 1910 and 1940 the average number of cigarettes smoked per day by men in the United States increased eight-fold, from about 0.5 per day to 4 per day. Between 1930 and 1960 the mortality from lung cancer (the number of deaths per 100,000 men per year) also increased about eight-fold, from 4 to 35. For women nearly similar increases in cigarette smoking and then in mortality from lung cancer occurred, with a delay of 25 years (Figure 2-1).

Lung cancer now causes 35 percent of the cancer deaths in men, more than any other kind of cancer. In 1978 close to 100,000 men and women in the United States died of lung cancer, for the most part because they smoked

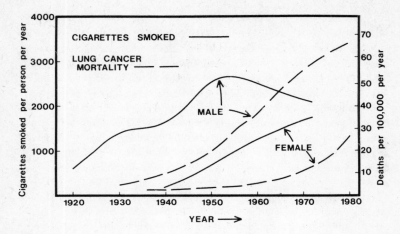

FIGURE 2-1
Mortality from lung cancer, which increased sharply about 25 years after smoking became popular, first among men and then among women.

cigarettes. Moreover, cigarette smokers have an increased probability at each age of dying from other forms of cancer and from heart disease and other diseases. The average cigarette smoker develops serious illnesses and dies 8 years earlier than the average non-smoker. On the average, each cigarette smoked decreases the life expectancy of the smoker by 10 minutes.

It is the delay of 15 to 30 years between exposure to the carcinogen, such as cigarette smoke, and the development of the recognizable cancer that worries many thoughtful people in the world today, people who can remember when cigarette smoking was a perfectly acceptable social habit with no suspicion of any danger. Since the Second World War we have lived in an increasingly "chemical" society, with plastics, pesticides, herbicides, artificial colors and flavors, food additives, and other chemicals to which the human body is not accustomed being manufactured on a gigantic scale. The Environmental Protection Agency has estimated that 60,000 chemicals are already in commercial use and that new ones are coming into use at the rate of 1000 a year. Many of these agents have been recognized to be carcinogenic and some of them have been banned. The tragedy is that it takes time to identify the carcinogens, however, and many people who are exposed to them before they are recognized and removed from the market will be caused to develop cancer that will appear only after the induction period of two or three decades.

High-energy radiation in all its forms—the alpha, beta, and gamma rays from radioactive substances, cosmic rays, x-rays, and even the ultraviolet rays in sunlight—also is carcinogenic. The high incidence of cancer in workers in the uranium industry has already been mentioned. Many of the women who from 1916 to 1924 painted the dials on watches and clocks with a radioactive paint and who brought a brush to a fine point by putting it between their lips, thus getting the radioactive radium or thorium into their bones, died later of bone cancer. The radioactive atomic nuclei liberated into the atmosphere by the test explosions of nuclear weapons (strontium 90, cesium 137, carbon 14, and others) are now present in every human being and continue to increase the incidence of cancer all over the world. Many of the scientists and physicians who worked with x-rays during the first decade or two after their discovery in 1896, until their carcinogenic power was discovered, developed cancer.

The natural exposure of people to high-energy radiation, part of which comes from cosmic rays and part from natural radioactivity (radium, potassium 40, tritium), varies from place to place but amounts on the average to about 100 milliroentgens per year. This unavoidable exposure causes genetic mutations that lead to the birth of infants with minor or gross congenital defects and also causes cancer. There is some uncertainty about how much cancer is caused by this amount of high-energy radiation, but we have confidence in the estimate made by Dr. Hardin B. Jones, late Professor of Medical Physics and Physiology in the University of California, Berkeley, who concluded that 9 percent of all cases of cancer are produced by it.

The average exposure of people in the United States to medical x-rays for diagnostic or therapeutic purposes is about the same, 100 milliroentgens per year, and medical x-rays may thus cause as many cancers as background radiation. Of course, it must be remembered that the use of x-rays in medical practice is of great value, and that the danger of genetic and somatic damage by the x-rays is one that often must be taken, although it should be kept to a minimum by taking care that the x-ray exposure is not made except when necessary and then not in amounts greater than necessary.

Continued exposure to sunlight of people whose skin is not strongly pigmented is related to an increased incidence of skin cancer. The conclusion that this increased incidence is caused by the ultraviolet rays in the sunlight has been made highly probable by careful studies of a similar effect of ultraviolet light on hairless mice.

Another apparent cause of cancer is heat. For example, some people in India who warm themselves by holding a pot of glowing coals under their clothes have an increased incidence of cancer of the skin in the area that is repeatedly heated by the hot pot.

These various "causes" of cancer represent in fact positive correlations: an increased incidence of cancer is observed to occur in the presence of some substance or circumstance so often as to force us to conclude that there is a cause-and-effect relationship. To understand cancer, however, we need to understand the molecular mechanisms that underlie it. There is no doubt that cancer cells are the normal cells of the body that have undergone a change. This change is heritable—it is passed on to the progeny of the original cancer cells. We know that the properties of the cells are determined primarily by the *genes,* the hereditary material present in the cell nuclei. A change in properties often means that a change has taken place in the nature of this material.

We now know a great deal about how these changes can take place. The genes are molecules of deoxyribonucleic acid, DNA. A gene is a linear sequence (a chain) of residues of four moderately small molecules, adenine (A), thymine (T), guanine (G), and cytosine (C), which are characteristic of somewhat larger molecules called nucleotides. The function of most genes is to direct the synthesis of a specific chain of amino acids, usually to form a protein molecule. There are twenty different kinds of these amino acids— glycine, alanine, lysine, and so on. A sequence of three nucleotides in the gene is needed to select each amino acid for the successive positions in the growing chain of a protein. Thus either the codeword AAA or AAG selects a molecule of the amino acid lysine, and either GAA or GAG selects a molecule of glutamic acid for the position in the chain.

One way in which the genetic character of a cell can be changed is by a point mutation in the DNA that constitutes one of its genes. It might happen that for some reason an error occurs in the genetic process of replication of a gene in the process of cell division, so that a daughter cell has inherited a gene with one nucleotide changed. For example, the sequence GAA, coding for glutamic acid, might have changed to AAA, coding for lysine. The gene might contain 438 "letters" (A, T, G, C) that make up 146 "words," thus defining a polypeptide chain of 146 amino-acid residues (the number actually present in the beta chains of the human hemoglobin molecule). The change of one of the 438 letters from G to A means that the protein chain has one amino-acid residue different in the daughter cell from that in the parent cell, in this case lysine in place of glutamic acid, with the other 145 amino-acid residues the same. This may seem to be a small change in the gene and in its product the protein, but it can be catastrophic to the human being. It is exactly this change that takes place in the gene for the beta chain of hemoglobin that causes the serious disease hemoglobin-C hemoglobinopathy. A similar point substitution, leading to replacement of glutamic acid by valine, leads to another serious disease, sickle-cell anemia. We can understand accordingly that a point mutation in a gene might confer upon a cell one of the properties that gives it malignancy.

A gene may also change in other ways. One way is deletion of some nucleotides. Thus in the above example the sequence GAA may simply be deleted; the corresponding chain would then contain only 145 amino acids, with the residue of glutamic acid missing.

It is astounding that the process of gene replication occurs with so few errors. Errors do occur, probably a few with every cell division among the 100,000 genes, each consisting of hundreds or even thousands of nucleotides, in the human cell. They may occur sometimes just because of thermal agitation of the atoms—the atomic vibrations that increase in amplitude with increase in temperature. This mechanism thus provides an explanation of the fact that the number of genetic mutations increases with increase in temperature, and also of the fact, noted above, that local heat can cause cancer.

Another way in which the nature of the cell's complement of DNA can change is through chromosomal abnormalities. The genes are clumped together into aggregates called chromosomes. In a normal human cell there are 46 chromosomes, each with 1000 to 3000 genes. Before a cell divides, each gene directs the manufacture of a duplicate of itself, so that each of the two daughter cells normally has its complement of 46 chromosomes. Sometimes, however, an error is made, such that one daughter cell contains 45 and the other contains 47 chromosomes. We can understand that to have only one of a pair of chromosomes could have a great effect on the properties of the cell. Each of the thousand or so genes on the chromosome would be present in the cell in only half the normal number, and presumably only half the normal amounts of their corresponding proteins would be synthesized. With 47 chromosomes we would expect many proteins to be synthesized at a rate 50 percent greater. Still larger deviations from the normal chromosome number also occur, as well as other abnormalities, such as the transfer of part of one chromosome to another, the inversion in direction of a part, or the loss of a part. Many congenital defects in human beings result from chromosomal abnormalities; for example, persons with Down's syndrome ("Mongolism") have three rather than two copies of one of the smallest chromosomes. Moreover, malignant tumors are observed to contain many cells that show chromosomal abnormalities. We can accept the idea that chromosomal abnormalities as well as gene mutations might confer upon cells the properties characteristic of malignancy.

Increased temperature, x-rays, gamma rays, ultraviolet rays, and many carcinogenic chemicals are known to cause gene mutations, chromosomal abnormalities, and other alterations in DNA content such as to give rise to the change in cell properties that make the cell malignant. In order to complete our understanding of cancer we now need only to answer the following questions:

What is cancer? What is a cancer cell?

We believe that these questions have a simple answer.

Cancer is a disease in which some of the cells of the body have undergone changes in their genetic material (DNA) such as to confer upon them the properties characteristic of cancer.

At first it may seem that in this statement we are just begging the question, just saying that cancer is cancer. But in fact there is content to our statement. There is no mystery about cancer. In a broad sense, we understand its nature and its causes. The body contains many normal cells. Their properties are determined by their DNA, as influenced to some extent by their environment. As these cells divide, some of the daughter cells may, but rather rarely, inherit somewhat different complements of DNA, because of gene mutation or chromosomal abnormality. Invasion by a virus might sometimes play a role. These changes in the genetic material usually result in cell death. However, when the cells have, by chance, acquired the set of properties characteristic of malignancy they become a cancer.

All that remains is to list the properties characteristic of malignancy. These are without doubt somewhat different for different kinds of cancer, but we have formulated the following basic set:

1. *The capacity for proliferation.* In normal tissues the cells are under some restraint on their growth to keep each part of the organism from encroaching on the other parts. Cancer cells have thrown off this restraint.

2. *The capacity for infiltration.* Cancer cells have developed the ability to attack normal tissues and to grow into them. This ability may involve several changes, such as those that lead to increased production not only of hyaluronidase and of collagenase, as mentioned in the preface, but also of other enzymes that can attack carbohydrates and proteins.

3. *The capacity to obtain increased amounts of nutrients and oxygen.* The rapid growth characteristic of cancers at some stages depends not only on the ability of the cells to divide rapidly but also on the availability of the required raw materials. For some cancers this result is achieved through the production and liberation into the surrounding tissues of a substance that increases diffusion and stimulates the growth of blood vessels into the cancer. Also some cancers cope with the problem of an insufficient supply of oxygen by making use of an alternative metabolic pathway ("fermentation") that requires less oxygen than the customary one.

From analysis of the rates at which cancer develops in both human beings and animals after they have been exposed to a carcinogenic agent or condition, it has been concluded that several different changes, usually five or six, in the properties of a cell or group of cells seem to take place before the malignancy comes into being. These several changes, the development of new properties, are of the kinds discussed above and in the earlier sections on precancer and cancer. Many observations about differences between cancers and normal tissues have been reported, usually involving the amount of some enzyme produced by the cells. Some of these differences are important to the malignancy, whereas others may be only incidental to the significant changes.

Now that we understand the enemy, we have the duty to conquer him.

Cancer is caused by agents and conditions that change the genetic material in the cells of our bodies. It is clearly sensible for us to strive to prevent these changes and thus to prevent cancer. High-energy radiation causes cancer; hence we should avoid being exposed to it—no unnecessary x-rays, no over-exposure to sunlight, no radioactive pollution from nuclear weapons tests or nuclear power plants. Many chemicals cause cancer; hence we should try to identify them and to ban them. Moreover, as will be pointed out later, vitamin C is a rather general detoxifying agent, and its proper use can help to protect us against carcinogenic chemicals, even those in tobacco smoke, although here the only sensible course is to stop smoking. Our normal tissues and organs fight the renegade malignancy; it is our duty to ourselves to help strengthen them in this fight, and there is evidence that vitamin C and other nutrients provide this strengthening influence.

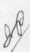

3

The Common Forms
of Human Cancer

It is possible to classify cancer into about 200 different types according to the kind of primary cell and its subsequent pattern of behavior. From an overall view, however, we must accept the idea that cancer is one disease, in the sense that the word describes a situation in which one cell, any cell, acquires the properties of unrestrained proliferation and invasiveness and is able to bequeath these properties to its descendants through countless generations. The result is cancer, no matter where the disease has arisen and irrespective of the degree of aggressiveness of its subsequent behavior.

In this chapter we shall describe some of the common forms of human cancer, their cause, if known, their likely symptoms, and their usual pattern of progression, including a brief summary of currently accepted regimes of treatment. In cancer "common things occur commonly," but great variation can occur in the dependence of incidence on age, in the symptomatology, and in the progression of the disease. These occasional bizarre presentations serve to emphasize that the great majority of human cancers follow a fairly predictable course. Before discussing the individual forms of cancer we shall define some common medical terms.

A *tumor* is any morbid (unhealthy) swelling: an abnormal mass of tissue arising from cells of pre-existent tissue. The word is often used as a synonym for the term *new growth* or *neoplasm*. The tumor or neoplasm may be benign or malignant.

A *benign* tumor consists of a steadily expanding mass of cells that do not infiltrate or invade surrounding tissues and never metastasize (form a similar lesion in a distant location). They tend to grow relatively slowly (although there are a few striking exceptions to this rule), to be well encapsulated, and to be relatively harmless except for local pressure effects. Thus a benign tumor of the breast may grow to a large size and prove to be an embarrassment to the patient, but pose no threat to her life, whereas an equally benign intracranial tumor growing within the rigid confines of the skull could cause severe neurological damage and even death from simple compression of the brain. All benign tumors carry some risk of eventual malignant change, and even though this risk is rather small their surgical removal is generally advisable.

A *malignant* tumor consists of a steadily expanding mass of cells that also infiltrate and invade surrounding tissues, metastasize, and, unless arrested, eventually overwhelm the patient. The general term cancer refers only to malignant tumors, and while the phrase *benign neoplasm* is accepted, common usage restricts the terms neoplasia and neoplastic disease to the malignant category.

Traditionally, malignant tumors are classified into three main categories, carcinomas, sarcomas, and miscellaneous others, according to their primary cell type and microscopic appearances. Because the fundamental behavioral characteristics of all cancers are essentially the same, such a classification is somewhat irrelevant. These terms are, however, so well established that some explanation is called for, to avoid unnecessary confusion.

Carcinomas are malignant tumors that arise from the cells of any covering membrane, either external, such as the skin, or internal, such as the linings of the ductal systems of the breast, the gastrointestinal tract, the pulmonary tract, the urogenital tract, or their associated glandular structures. Because such covering surfaces are the first to be exposed to carcinogenic influences, carcinomas account for more than 90 percent of all malignancies. The term *adenocarcinoma* indicates that the tumor has arisen from some glandular structure and has retained some semblance of glandular formation even in malignancy. In contrast, and as explained earlier, an *anaplastic carcinoma* is a tumor so primitive that it has retained no trace of structural organization. One type of carcinoma is so common as to merit the special label *squamous-cell epithelioma*. This term refers to a tumor of moderate malignancy still retaining the microscopic characteristics of its tissue of origin, the squamous epithelium of the skin, lining of the esophagus, or other membrane.

Sarcomas are tumors of the supporting tissues, such as the bony skeleton *(osteogenic sarcoma)*, cartilage *(chondrosarcoma)*, muscle *(myosarcoma)*, fibrous tissue *(fibrosarcoma)*, joint surfaces *(synoviosarcoma)*, and fat *(liposarcoma)*. Sarcomas comprise less than 5 percent of all malignant tumors.

The remaining malignant tumors arise neither from covering membranes nor supporting structures, but from individual highly specialized cells in the tissues. Although such "miscellaneous others" account for a relatively small proportion of all malignancies, the category includes a wide variety of individual tumor types, ranging from the malignant melanomas of skin and other tissues, through the leukemias and the lymphomas of the reticulo-endothelial system, to the gliomas and meningiomas of the brain and central nervous system, and very many more. The usual behavior pattern of most of these tumors will be described later in this chapter.

The precise identification of an individual tumor yields very valuable prognostic information. Exceptions may occur, but the great majority of tumors tend to behave in a predictable manner, depending upon their cellular appearance and organ of origin. Some individual cancers will now be described.

CANCER OF THE SKIN

There are three main types of cancer of the skin.

The most common and the least dangerous is the *basal cell carcinoma* or *rodent ulcer*. This cancer is caused by excessive exposure to ultraviolet radiation, commonly by sunlight, and is therefore seen most frequently in people of Northern European stock living in areas of high solar intensity, such as the American South and West, South Africa, and Australia. For the same reason it is more common on the face and hands than elsewhere. It forms an extremely slow-growing skin nodule that eventually ulcerates with a characteristically pearly margin. It may take several years to reach a diameter of even óne quarter of an inch and, although locally invasive, it never metastasizes. It is the easiest of all cancers to cure, and for this reason is often left out of gross cancer statistics. It can be cured by simple surgical excision, by low-dose X-irradiation to the area, or even by the brief local application of intense cold. After any of these simple treatments local recurrence is almost unknown, but similar lesions may occur elsewhere, so continued surveillance is essential.

The next most common form of skin cancer is *squamous-cell epithelioma,* which grows rapidly, forming a raised protruding ulcer with a distinctly hard margin, and which spreads predominantly to the regional lymph nodes. This type of cancer is also most common on exposed parts of the skin, but it can occur elsewhere. It can also be caused by local heat and chronic irritation, as on the lips and tongue of pipe smokers and trumpet players. It is usually curable by surgical excision of the local lesion with or without excision of the regional lymph nodes, if they are involved. Such lesions are also fairly responsive to radiotherapy, and the overall cure rates are reasonably good whether surgery, radiotherapy, or some combination of the two is used. However, some patients with squamous epithelioma die from widespread metastases in spite of conventional treatment. As in many other cancer situations, the chance of this outcome can be diminished by early diagnosis and treatment. In general, squamous epitheliomas are fairly resistant to the cancer chemotherapeutic drugs available at the present time.

The most dangerous form of skin cancer is *malignant melanoma (malignant pigmented mole)*. This cancer may arise in a previously benign pigmented mole or birthmark, which suddenly starts to enlarge and to bleed, or it may arise as a totally new lesion. It also appears to have a causative relationship to sunlight, and it tends to be a disease of much younger age groups than those usually afflicted with the other two forms of skin cancer. It is usually a highly invasive tumor with early entry into the lymphatic and circulatory systems, and a correspondingly poor prognosis. The tumor is usually radiation-resistant, and responses to chemotherapy tend to be minimal. If the tumor is still confined to its primary site prompt surgical excision can often result in cure. When the tumor has already spread to the regional lymph nodes, local excision plus removal of these lymph nodes can still result in cure, but the chances of success diminish rapidly with the passage of time. There is really no cure for disseminated malignant melanoma, but there is at least one ray of hope. Spontaneous regression has been reported to occur in quite a number of far-advanced cases of this disease, and many such patients are now being treated by immunotherapy in the hope that a powerful immune reaction would overwhelm the tumor. So far as we are aware no genuine sustained cure has yet been obtained by such methods, but some temporary remissions have been recorded. These results will no doubt improve as techniques become more refined. We feel strongly that this is precisely the situation where immuno-stimulation and high ascorbate intake could work together and effect some improvement in what can only be described as an extremely dismal clinical situation.

CANCERS OF THE NASAL SINUSES, THROAT, AND PHARYNX

Cancers of the nasal sinuses, throat, and pharynx, three relatively rare but particularly unpleasant forms of cancer, have some causal relationship to smoking and to the repeated inhalation of toxic fumes in certain industrial situations. They tend to cause trouble more by local infiltration than by distant metastases. They declare their presence by some interference with normal function, by local pain, nosebleeds, or hoarseness. They tend to be in anatomically inaccessible situations, making surgery both difficult and mutilating. Fortunately the majority are fairly radio-sensitive, and radiotherapy is usually the treatment of choice. A comparatively rare but intriguing form of malignancy that occurs predominantly in this anatomical situation is *Burkitt's lymphoma* of equatorial Africa, a highly malignant tumor of children caused by a combination of an insect-borne virus and chronic malarial infestation, and confined to very precise geographical locations where these causative factors exist in the environment. It responds quite dramatically to either radiotherapy or cytotoxic chemotherapy.

CANCER OF THE LARYNX

There is some evidence that cancer of the vocal cords is more common in vocalists, be they actors or singers, than in other people. It makes its presence felt at an early stage by hoarseness, and at that stage can often be cured by relatively minor local surgery. For more advanced growths radiotherapy records a fair proportion of successes, but in radio-resistant situations removal of the whole larynx is required. This is not a life-threatening operation, but it leaves the patient incapable of normal speech. This severe handicap is counterbalanced by the fact that the cure rate is very high—few patients die from laryngeal cancer.

CANCER OF THE ESOPHAGUS

Cancer of the esophagus is relatively rare in the Western world, but has a high incidence in certain parts of the Middle East and Turkey, where dietary habits involve the frequent swallowing of very hot drinks, suggesting that this cancer may be causally related to repeated local injury to the esophageal lining. It also has a particularly high incidence in certain provinces of China where traditional methods of grain storage result in a high carcinogenic nitrosamine content of the grain. It tends in the Western world to be a disease of males, and is notably more common in American blacks than in American whites. The symptoms are usually clear-cut—mechanical difficulty in swallowing, with a sensation of food sticking in the gullet, and as the illness progresses difficulty in swallowing even liquids, regurgitation of clean undigested food, and fairly rapid weight loss from simple starvation. The overall results of conventional treatments are quite abysmal, with less than 4 percent of such patients surviving five years after first diagnosis. The tumor tends to spread to the liver, but the patient usually dies from starvation rather than from widespread metastatic disease. The methods of treatment available are surgical removal of the affected segment of the esophagus, a difficult procedure involving a high degree of risk, and accurately directed radiotherapy, which occasionally proves to be remarkably successful. There is a lighter side to this dismal picture. The disease tends to be one of the elderly, and the tumor itself tends to be relatively slow growing, causing more mischief from local obstruction than from its spread. The mechanical problem can be overcome by the simple palliative procedure of intubation—the insertion of a semi-rigid plastic tube through the tumor. This minor operation, which can often be done through an esophagoscope without the need for any external incision, completely relieves the patient's swallowing difficulties, and he may live thereafter in relative comfort for many months or even some years.

CANCER OF THE STOMACH

The age-standardized mortality from stomach cancer in the United States has decreased by 75 percent since 1930. There is circumstantial evidence that this welcome decrease reflects the increased use of domestic refrigerators and the decreased reliance on nitrates to preserve bacon and other meat foods. Nitrates react in the acid environment of the stomach with the contents of many foods to form highly carcinogenic nitrosamines, which act on their first contact, the stomach lining. The removal of nitrates from foods reduces this danger. It is also well established that vitamin C prevents nitrosamine formation, and it is reasonable to assume that the trend towards an increasing consumption of fruits and vegetables rich in vitamin C is also responsible for the downturn in the incidence of stomach cancer. The mortality from stomach cancer in Japan is the highest in the world, being eight times that in the United States. This high value is partially related to nitrates, but more so to a heavy nutritional dependency upon smoked and broiled foods, which are rich in carcinogenic hydrocarbons, and to the widespread consumption of a prized national delicacy, bracken fern. (It is interesting to note that cattle grazing on poor pastures in the North of Scotland, where bracken abounds, also have a very high incidence of stomach cancer.) Other etiological factors operating in stomach cancer are some apparently strong genetic influences—a history of close relatives with this form of cancer confers an added risk, although common familial nutritional patterns may be at work there. Another predisposing factor is a preceding history of atrophic gastritis, which often makes itself known years before the appearance of the tumor by the development of pernicious (megaloblastic) anemia.

The characteristic symptoms of stomach cancer are an abrupt loss of appetite, such that even the very sight of food is nauseating, progressive anemia from gastric blood loss, increasing lassitude out of proportion to the degree of anemia, difficulty in swallowing if the tumor is in the high stomach, obstructive vomiting if the tumor is in the low stomach, and, almost invariably, sharp weight loss. The tumor can sometimes be palpated through the relaxed abdominal wall. The diagnosis is confirmed by an x-ray examination following a barium-compound meal that outlines the stomach and permits examination of its contour for tumor irregularity and differences in motility, and if necessary by gastroscopy, the swallowing of a flexible fiberoptic telescope that enables the physician to inspect the interior of the empty stomach.

Gastric cancers are almost always carcinomas, but occasional myosarcomas occur, with a slightly better prognosis. Both types of tumor spread primarily to the regional lymph nodes, which can be surgically removed, and thence to the liver whence, unless in the very exceptional circumstance of a solitary operable metastasis, they cannot be removed, and the situation is incurable.

The technical problems associated with the surgical treatment of stomach cancer will be mentioned in a later chapter, but in the present stage of our knowledge surgery provides the best chance of control by conventional methods. Radiotherapy has nothing to offer in this situation, and although chemotherapy is frequently used, there is very real doubt whether it is of any value. On the other hand, there is some evidence, discussed in later chapters, that ascorbate therapy offers significant promise of value for control of this form of cancer.

CANCER OF THE DUODENUM AND THE SMALL INTESTINE

Cancer of the duodenum is almost unknown, and this local immunity when compared to the frequent occurrence in the contiguous stomach is an intriguing feature of this strange disease. Cancer of the whole small intestine is also remarkably rare, and this relative immunity is thought to be due to the fast transit times of ingested foods with their associated carcinogens, minimizing any local exposure. This form of cancer often announces itself quite abruptly as an acute intestinal obstruction with frequent colicky abdominal pains, rapidly increasing abdominal distension, and profuse vomiting—a situation requiring emergency surgery, during which this comparatively rare diagnosis is established. The surgical problem is handled by carrying out a wedge resection (Figure 3-1).

This standard operative procedure removes the tumor, an adequate margin of healthy intestine above and below it, and a wedge of the mesentery contain-

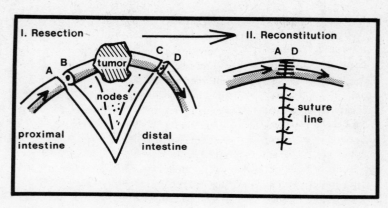

FIGURE 3-1
The operation of wedge resection for intestinal tumors.

ing the related lymph nodes. If the primary tumor is resectable it must be removed or at least bypassed to relieve the urgent symptoms. A variety of histological types of tumor occur in this area, and none can be treated by radiotherapy. If the tumor is a carcinoma and liver or other irresectable metastases are present, chemotherapy is of only dubious value. If however, the tumor is a sarcoma, and in particular a lymphosarcoma, chemotherapy can prove to be highly beneficial.

CANCERS OF THE COLON AND RECTUM

Cancer of the large intestine is far more common than cancer of the small intestine, because transit time is progressively slowed by fluid reabsorption to form a semi-solid stool, thus increasing contact exposure to fecal carcinogens. Cancer of the large intestine is also much more common in the Western world than in less sophisticated communities. There is circumstantial evidence that the lack of fiber roughage in sophisticated diets is responsible for this difference. A high proportion of indigestible cellulose fiber is thought to lead to healthy bowel evacuation; removal of this roughage by modern food-processing technology results in small stools, chronic constipation, and prolonged exposure of the colo-rectal mucosa to fecal carcinogens. These have been identified in part as nitrosamines, produced from ingested nitrate and bacterial action in a constipated large bowel, and it has been established that their formation can be blocked by an adequate intake of vitamin C. Moreover, a good intake of vitamin C acts as a laxative, and thus decreases the time of exposure of the colon and rectum to the action of the fecal carcinogens.

There are some other predisposing factors in colo-rectal cancer. Patients with familial colonic polyposis (multiple benign colonic tumors) almost invariably develop colonic cancer at some time in their adult life. Patients with uncontrolled ulcerative colitis for 10 or more years very frequently succumb to colonic cancer, and because of the very long duration of bowel symptoms the transition to malignancy is usually almost impossible to perceive. Vitamin C ingestion has been shown to induce regression in colonic polyposis, and it is reasonable to assume that it would also afford some protection in ulcerative colitis, although we are not aware of any specific studies in the latter area.

The symptoms of large-bowel cancer depend upon whether the tumor is in the right colon, the left colon, or the rectum.

In the right colon (the cecum, the ascending colon, and the proximal transverse colon, Figure 3-2) the bowel caliber is relatively large and the bowel contents are fairly fluid, and therefore obstructive symptoms rarely occur. The usual symptoms of a cancer of the right colon are a rather vague blend of anemia from blood loss from the tumor, weight loss from the systemic toxemia of an ulcerated tumor constantly bathed in liquid feces, and often very little else. Such a vague symptomatology is often confused with that of cancer of the stomach, and in such circumstances it is customary to request a "full G.I. series," that is, a complete radiological examination of the stomach, small intestine, and large intestine. This examination will locate the tumor, and the primary treatment is then by surgery, in the form of a wedge resection, but because of local anatomical considerations somewhat more elaborate than the simple procedure already depicted. Such tumors metastasize in the first instance to their regional lymph nodes in the related mesentery (operable) and thence to the liver (incurable).

In the left colon (the distal transverse colon, the descending colon, and, the most common site of all, the sigmoid colon, Figure 3-2), the bowel diameter becomes progressively smaller and the fecal content becomes more solid, and hence obstructive symptoms predominate. These may declare themselves as alternating periods of constipation and "overflow" diarrhea, or they may seize a patient with little or no prior warning as the acute surgical emergency of large-bowel obstruction. In the former circumstances the diagnosis can usually be established with relative ease by use of conventional radiography and if necessary by colonoscopy. In the latter circumstance emergency surgery is usually required and the diagnosis is established at operation. The treatment is again by wedge resection, the extent of the resection being governed by the blood supply and associated lymph-node drainage at different sites.

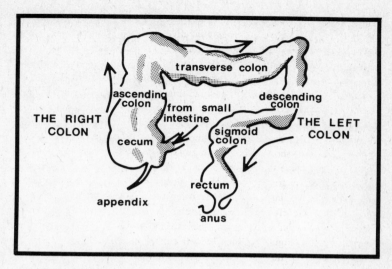

FIGURE 3-2
The anatomy of the colon and rectum.

Because tumors of the right colon tend to present themselves insidiously and tumors of the left colon more dramatically, by the time the diagnosis is reached liver metastases tend to be more common in the former group, with a correspondingly poorer overall prognosis. Radiotherapy is quite useless in colonic cancer, because to irradiate such an intra-abdominal target would result in unacceptable damage to the normal tissues. At the present time chemotherapy is widely used in inoperable situations, and although some useful retardation of tumor growth may sometimes be achieved the response is highly unpredictable and the side effects are so disagreeable as to make the value of the treatment doubtful.

Cancer of the rectum grows in an easily distensible part of the lower bowel, and accordingly obstructive symptoms virtually never occur. Instead the symptoms are of bowel irregularity, blood in the feces, and a constant urge to defecate, together with tenesmus, the feeling of incomplete bowel evacuation because of the presence of this often quite bulky tumor. The diagnosis is easily established by simple digital examination. The tumor tends to grow relatively slowly and to spread more by local infiltration into the bladder and other pelvic organs than by metastasizing widely. When metastases are present the usual first site is in the liver. The only effective treatment is by surgical removal by the standard operative procedure known as abdomino-perineal excision. This removes the whole lower sigmoid and lymph nodes, the rectum, and the anus, and leaves the patient with a permanent colostomy. (Colostomy care is beyond the scope of this book, but it may be said that with modern colostomy appliances and some dietary adjustments the colostomy patient can live an active and busy life with no social problems.)

Preoperative radiotherapy is of some value in rectal cancer in shrinking the size of the tumor mass and rendering border-line situations operable. It is of undoubted value in controlling any recurrences in the perineal scar. Because rectal cancers tend to be relatively slow-growing, chemotherapy is of very limited value.

Cancer of the anus is usually a squamous epithelioma, and, like similar tumors elsewhere, it can often be cured by radiotherapy alone. Ascorbate therapy has recently been reported to be effective (Chapter 22).

CANCER OF THE PANCREAS

No obvious cause for cancer of the pancreas has been identified; it is, however, about twice as common in cigarette smokers as in non-smokers. The bile duct, which conveys bile from the liver to the intestine, passes through the head of the pancreas, and a pancreatic cancer at that site, which is the most common, makes itself known by compression of the bile duct, causing painless progressively deepening jaundice (from the retention of bile pigments in the bloodstream), intense skin itch (from the retention of bile salts in the bloodstream), the passage of pale bulky stools (from the absence of bile and impaired enzymatic digestion), and dark urine (from the spillover of bile pigment). As mentioned in Chapter 5, surgical removal of such a pancreatic cancer is technically possible, but, being a matter of appreciable risk and with considerable post-operative morbidity, it is seldom performed. The tumor spreads to adjacent lymph nodes and thence to the liver, but if the disease is not treated death usually occurs from obstructive liver failure long before this metastatic spread. There is a bright side to this picture. The tumor is usually rather slow growing, and it occurs predominantly in the elderly. The obstructive jaundice can be relieved by a relatively minor by-pass operation, allowing the jaundice to clear, and the patient may then enjoy reasonably good health for many months and sometimes years.

Cancer of the body of the pancreas, not obstructing the bile duct, is notoriously difficult to diagnose because the symptoms are so vague. The usual story is of diminishing appetite and loss of weight, with later constant upper abdominal discomfort and backache. In the authors' opinion this form of cancer is untreatable by any known conventional method of therapy.

CANCER OF THE GALLBLADDER

Gallstones are comparatively common and cancer of the gallbladder is relatively rare, but cancer never occurs in a gallbladder without stones first being present. Familial and nutritional factors are involved in gallstone formulation, producing the classical "fair, fertile, fat, and forty" stereotype. Recently, however, there has been a marked increase in the incidence of gallstones in younger women, and there is fairly strong circumstantial evidence linking this increased incidence with the widespread use of oral contraceptives. Thus by a circuitous route today's use of oral contraceptives may result in an increase in gallbladder cancer some 15 or 20 years hence. The relationship between gallstones and subsequent gallbladder cancer is so strong that even symptomless gallstones should be prophylactically removed. Only very early cases of gallbladder cancer are surgically curable, because the tumor readily infiltrates into the adjacent liver, rendering the whole situation irresectable. Radiotherapy and chemotherapy have nothing to offer in such circumstances.

CANCER OF THE LIVER

Primary cancer of the liver is very rare in the Western world but is common in many of the developing countries, where chronic liver damage from long-continued protein starvation is still a harsh fact of life. In the Western world liver cancer is usually associated with the chronic liver damage of alcoholic cirrhosis. Vinyl chloride, the building block of the plastic polyvinyl chloride (PVC), has caused a rare form of primary liver cancer among workers exposed to it, and there is some concern that the PVC widely used in food packaging and in domestic plumbing may be liberating traces of the dangerous vinyl chloride and that years from now we may witness a sharp increase in this form of cancer.

In only very rare instances is a primary liver cancer so situated and so localized that its surgical removal is possible. If the tumor is rapidly growing and anaplastic, some response, but not cure, can be anticipated from chemotherapy.

The liver is by far the most common site of secondary metastatic tumors spreading from primaries elsewhere, particularly primary tumors of the gastrointestinal system. Their presence usually indicates an incurable situation. Malignant liver enlargement can usually be felt by the physician, and the size and location of individual liver metastases can be visualized and measured by ultrasound, isotope liver scan, or computerized axial tomography (CAT-scan).

CANCER OF THE KIDNEY

There are two quite different types of cancer that affect the kidney.

The rarer of the two is known as *transitional-cell papillomatosis,* a type of tumor that may arise anywhere in the special endothelial lining of the kidney, ureter, or bladder. If the disease is still confined to one kidney, the treatment is by the surgical removal of that kidney, but this form of malignancy tends to be multifocal; that is, similar tumors tend to appear elsewhere throughout the urinary collecting system. This will be discussed more fully below under cancer of the bladder.

The common kidney cancer is an adenocarcinoma, also known by its traditional name *hypernephroma.* While every variant is possible, kidney cancer tends to be a cancer of moderate growth rate and to be a disease of the middle aged and elderly. In the human no causative factors have yet been identified, but identical tumors can be produced in some experimental animals by large doses of estrogens. The tumor expands steadily in the affected kidney and may reach a considerable size before any symptoms appear. The classical symptoms are hematuria (the passing of blood in the urine), with or without dull dragging discomfort in the affected loin. Hematuria has many other causes, but the possibility of malignancy must always be excluded by thorough investigation. The diagnosis can be confirmed by simple radiography and the treatment is by surgical removal of the whole tumor-bearing kidney.

As untreated or unsuspected disease progresses, the tumor enters the renal (kidney) vein and widespread skeletal and pulmonary metastases are the general rule. In these circumstances radiotherapy and chemotherapy are of little value, but some patients obtain temporary remissions from hormonal therapy.

Renal carcinomas demonstrate a few unusual characteristics. In most cancers the recognition of even one distant metastasis indicates that many other metastases are already present. A solitary metastasis can occur in a renal carcinoma, however, and in such a circumstance surgical removal of the diseased kidney with its solitary metastasis is justifiable. Sometimes such a treatment is carried out inadvertently; it is not uncommon for a symptomless and unsuspected renal tumor to declare itself by the appearance of a solitary metastasis in the lung, a bone, or the brain, and under such a circumstance it may be removed by a thoracic surgeon, an orthopedic surgeon, or a neurosurgeon under the impression that he is dealing with a primary tumor. Microscopic examination establishes the correct diagnosis, and if no other obvious metastases are present the correct treatment is then to remove the diseased kidney. A few cases of renal cancer are on record in which removal of the primary tumor in the presence of known metastases has resulted in regression and disappearance of the metastases. This, it must be emphasized, is a very rare occurrence, but the fact that it can happen at all is remarkable.

CANCER OF THE BLADDER

Cancers of the bladder lining (and of the renal collecting systems mentioned above) range all the way from almost innocuous benign warty growths through lesions of increasing malignancy to solid ulcerating deeply invasive tumors. During an illness with bladder cancer, which may extend over very many years, there is a relentless progression from the benign to the more malignant end of the scale. The disease is multifocal in origin, meaning that the whole mucosa from kidney to bladder is unstable and in a pre-malignant condition. This means that even if one tumor at point A in the bladder is successfully treated, similar lesions are very likely to appear at points B or C, and that continued surveillance is essential. The association between exposure to certain industrial chemicals and the development of bladder cancer is very well established. Also there is an increased incidence of bladder cancer in heavy tobacco smokers and heavy coffee drinkers as well as in certain persons with some inborn error of tryptophan metabolism. All these circumstances, occupational, social, and metabolic, result in the excretion of chemical carcinogens in the urine. There are also other urinary carcinogens that have still to be identified.

Bladder cancer usually makes its presence known by hematuria. Other symptoms are increased frequency and urgency of micturition (urination), resulting from diminished bladder capacity, and finally local pain. The condition is diagnosed, assessed, and in early cases treated by cystoscopy—the passage of a fiberoptic telescope along the urethra into the bladder under anesthesia.

Small lesions and lesions that are still clearly towards the benign end of the spectrum can be treated satisfactorily by cystoscopic electrocoagulation. Larger lesions may require that this procedure be carried out through the open bladder, or, if the tumor is invasive but still comparatively localized, that the whole tumor-bearing segment of the bladder be removed (partial cystectomy). For still larger and more deeply invasive tumors, the first choice of treatment is usually megavoltage radiotherapy, which, although individually rather unpredictable in response, can often be remarkably effective and curative in this situation. If all these methods fail to control the disease, the final choice is total removal of the urinary bladder (total cystectomy in the female, total cysto-prostatectomy in the male). Such a procedure clearly requires some form of urinary diversion, either by implanting the ureters to drain into the sigmoid colon or by implanting them into an artificial bladder formed from an isolated loop of small intestine opening through the abdominal wall. The former procedure subjects the patient to the risks of renal infections and biochemical disturbances, while the latter necessitates the constant wearing of an ileostomy bag. Bladder cancer is relatively slow growing and tends to cause symptoms more by infiltration of adjacent organs than by distant metastases. Total cystectomy is by any standards major surgery, with an appreciable operative risk and considerable post-operative morbidity. However, the alternative, to leave such a patient untreated, condemns him to a particularly cruel and miserable death.

Urologists at Tulane University (Schlegel et al., 1967, 1969, 1975) have shown that the regular ingestion of high levels of vitamin C neutralizes many bladder carcinogens, and furthermore can diminish very significantly bladder tumor recurrence and progression. The widespread adoption of such a simple measure could reduce much human suffering and perhaps abolish altogether the need for such procedures as total cystectomy.

CANCER OF THE PROSTATE GLAND

The prostate is the gland surrounding the bladder neck in males. Enlargement of the prostate gland is a very common accompaniment of the aging process. Most of these prostatic problems are perfectly benign, but a fraction are malignant, and this fraction increases with advancing years. The early symptoms of both illnesses are identical—obstruction to the voiding of urine, with increasing frequency of urination, nocturia (need to urinate during the night), and a feeling of incomplete emptying of the bladder. This may progress in both types of disorder to a complete inability to void urine, requiring emergency relief by use of a catheter. Digital rectal examination can usually distinguish benign from malignant prostatic enlargements with fair confidence and some simple biochemical tests can be used to confirm the diagnosis. The treatment of benign prostatic enlargement is surgery if the symptoms merit such a step. The treatment of cancer of the prostate is by estrogens (Chapter 8). Prostatic cancer tends to metastasize almost exclusively to the bony skeleton, with local pain over each such lesion. In the great majority of patients estrogens will bring rapid relief of pain and result in the regression of the bone metastases. For those patients who fail to respond to estrogens, and who tend to belong to a predominantly younger group, treatment is less satisfactory, although if the tumor is highly anaplastic some response from both radiotherapy and chemotherapy can be anticipated. We have observed some benefit in such patients in the relief of bone pain by regular high intakes of vitamin C, but there have been too few patients in this category to allow us to make any specific statement about prolongation of survival time.

TESTICULAR CANCER

There are many different testicular tumor types, seminomas and teratomas. On the whole, testicular cancers tend to be highly aggressive and to occur predominantly in relatively young men. The precise cause is unknown, but these cancers are far commoner in the atrophic (shrunken) testicle than in the normal testicle. Thus this form of cancer is far commoner in undescended testicles and in men with azoospermia and other subfertility problems than in others. The early symptoms are simply a steady heavy enlargement of the affected testicle. The treatment is by surgical removal of the diseased organ, usually followed by radiation to the para-aortic lymph nodes, to which such tumors first metastasize. If the disease has not been arrested, further spread takes place characteristically to the lungs and then body-wide. Until comparatively recently such a situation was virtually hopeless. At the time of the writing of this book the new cytotoxic drug cis-platinum (cis-dimethylplatinum dichloride) has been reported to induce dramatic and complete regression in a number of such patients, although it is too early yet to say whether these responses will result in permanent cures. Nevertheless this is an encouraging development, not only for the management of testicular cancer of young men, but as knowledge and experience increase, perhaps for other cancers as well.

CANCER OF THE OVARY

There are many types of ovarian tumors, and their behavior can range from virtually benign to the most malignant. Many of these tumors are cystic (forming a cavity) and grow rapidly in size, but it should be noted that sheer size bears no relationship to the degree of malignancy. The initial symptoms may be no more than an increasing abdominal distension, or may arise from pressure on adjacent pelvic organs, giving rise to bladder and bowel irregularity and a "bearing down" sensation. The initial treatment of choice is removal of the tumor, which must include removal of the womb and the other ovary because such tumors tend to be bilateral. These tumors spread predominantly by seeding to the liver and throughout the abdominal cavity, producing a massive accumulation of fluid ("ascites"). Depending upon the precise histology (the more anaplastic, the more rapidly growing), some ovarian cancers show a good response to either radiotherapy or chemotherapy. In advanced cases with recurrent tense ascites requiring repeated aspiration of the ascitic fluid for patient comfort, some retardation can be anticipated from the intraperitoneal injection of a cytotoxic drug, and Thio-Tepa is usually used for this purpose.

CANCER OF THE BODY OF THE UTERUS (ENDOMETRIAL CANCER)

Cancer of the body of the uterus is most common in women around the menopause. The precise cause is unknown but it is likely to be related to hormonal change. Some authorities have expressed concern that the prolonged use of oral contraceptives, which maintain the lining of the uterus, the endometrium, in a prolonged state of pseudo-pregnancy, might have a delayed carcinogenic effect, but to date there is not much evidence to support such a fear. Endometrial cancer makes its presence known by menstrual irregularity, post-menopausal bleeding, and abnormally heavy menstrual periods. These warning signs appear early, and the diagnosis is easily established by diagnostic uterine curettage. The treatment is by hysterectomy, resulting in a high rate of cure. In patients whose disease has already spread beyond the limits of surgery, about 40 percent will obtain a useful remission from appropriate hormonal treatment.

CANCER OF THE UTERINE CERVIX

Cancer of the uterine cervix (or neck), a very common form of female cancer, has been described by some as a venereal disease. The reason for this astonishing statement, which is, of course, untrue, is that it rarely occurs in nuns, that it occurs more frequently in the sexually promiscuous, and that its incidence increases as the age at first intercourse decreases. It is also relatively rare in Jewish women and among other ethnic groups where male circumcision is traditionally practiced. This is the form of cancer that cervical cytology (the Pap smear) is designed to detect in its early stages, and public health programs throughout the world have shown this procedure with proper treatment when indicated to be a most effective prophylactic measure. Such a technique is particularly valuable in cancer of the cervix, in which, because of lack of symptoms, quite advanced disease may be present without the most fastidious patient even being aware of it. A Pap smear can detect anything from pre-malignant change to frank cancer. All suspicious smears merit a full gynecological examination and usually a cone biopsy of the cervix. If no true invasiveness is seen, no further treatment is required. If true invasiveness is present, or obvious cancer is found on examination, the choice of treatment lies between total hysterectomy, Wertheim's hysterectomy (a more extensive procedure involving the removal of the pelvic lymph nodes), and radiotherapy. In patients with the disease in an early stage the results are equally good whatever method is chosen. Surgery is usually required in more advanced cases. Cancer of the cervix, like most other deep pelvic cancers, tends to grow comparatively slowly and to cause more havoc and distress by local infiltration than by the spread of distant metastases. Thus in very advanced cases the bladder and rectum may become involved, with very distressing local symptoms even in the absence of any life-threatening metastases elsewhere. In such a circumstance extensive surgery (exenteration, the removal of all involved organs) is required. The prime object of such a major operative procedure is not so much to gain a cure, although this can still occur in a significant proportion of these patients, as to gain symptomatic relief from pain, total urinary and fecal incontinence, and the like. The widespread availability and utilization of the Pap-smear technique should soon abolish forever such tragic human situations.

CANCER OF THE LUNG

The relationship between cigarette smoking and lung cancer needs hardly be stressed here (see Chapter 2) except to note that lung cancer can also affect lifelong non-smokers. It is also much more common in people living in urban than in rural areas and in countries with cold damp climates, where chronic bronchitis is rife. Chronic exposure to dust inhalation in many industrial processes, particularly in the mining industries, is also a causative factor.

Like smoking, lung cancer is predominantly a disease of men, but the incidence in women is rising steadily (Chapter 2). The illness may arise quite suddenly in someone in apparent good health and typically in his fifties, or it may be superimposed insidiously after a long history of chronic bronchitis and emphysema, typically in a patient in his seventies. The symptoms are often very vague, with chronic cough, the spitting up of blood, increasing breathlessness, and sharp weight loss. A common presentation is "pneumonia" or "pleurisy" that fails to respond to treatment. Very often the first indication of this disease is some metastatic manifestation, such as bone pain from a secondary tumor deposit, hoarseness from compression of the recurrent laryngeal nerve, or headache and irrational behavior from a brain metastasis. The diagnosis is usually very obvious on simple chest x-ray and if any doubt remains it can be confirmed by bronchoscopy and biopsy.

The only really curative treatment is early and adequate surgery. Each lung consists of several lobes. If the tumor is far out from the main lung root, it is sometimes possible to remove only the affected lobe (to carry out a lobectomy), with relatively minor residual respiratory impairment. If the tumor is more centrally situated, it may be possible to treat it by removal of the whole lung (pneumonectomy). This, of course, results in a 50-percent reduction in respiratory volume, but in time the remaining lung can compensate quite remarkably. If the tumor is more central still, invading the vital structures of the mediastinum (the septum between the lungs), the situation is inoperable. Unfortunately, the great majority of lung-cancer victims are inoperable when first diagnosed, either because of the site of the primary tumor or because metastases are already present.

Treatment of these inoperable situations is most unsatisfactory. Radiotherapy and chemotherapy are often used and, although occasional worthwhile responses are recorded, such beneficial responses are the exception to the general rule. The overall cure rates in cancer of the lung are extremely poor, and the survival time from the date of diagnosis until the date of death is usually comparatively short and measurable in months. Some benefit from ascorbate therapy has been observed (see later chapters).

A cancer of the pleural covering of the lung is known as a mesothelioma. This somewhat rare form of cancer, which can also arise in the peritoneal lining of the abdomen, is usually associated with asbestos exposure. It tends to be highly aggressive and to pursue a brisk downhill course. It is virtually untreatable by any conventional method of therapy.

CANCER OF THE BREAST

The precise cause of cancer of the breast, the commonest of all cancers in women, is unknown, although it is certain that hormonal factors are involved. Cancer of the breast is more common in spinsters than in married women, more common in those who have never lactated than in those who have, and least common of all in those who have breast-fed a number of children. It can occur at almost any age, with a peak incidence around the menopause. The diagnosis is made by the discovery of a painless lump in the breast, with later dimpling of the overlying skin and retraction of the nipple. The disease spreads to the axillary lymph nodes and sometimes to the intrathoracic lymph nodes, and then eventually by blood-borne dissemination predominantly to the skeleton and to the lung. All rates of growth can occur, but by and large this is often a comparatively slow growing tumor, and recurrences as long as 30 years after primary treatment are by no means unknown. Thus the conventional characteristic time defining a cancer "cure"—a patient alive and well with no evidence of active disease five years after primary treatment—has to be extended in considering cancer of the breast. A patient with breast cancer still confined to the breast has an excellent chance of long-term survival following simple local surgery. The achievements and the problems associated with treating patients with more advanced disease will be discussed in some later chapters, as well as the observations about ascorbate therapy.

Approximately one in every one hundred breast cancers occurs in men. The symptoms, the signs, and the methods of treatment are essentially the same, but the outlook is somewhat poorer because of the increased likelihood of early intrathoracic lymph-node spread.

THE SARCOMAS

An *osteogenic sarcoma* is a highly malignant tumor that almost always arises in the growing ends of long bones. Thus its incidence is virtually confined to growing teenagers, and the most common site is at the knee. The cause is unknown but there frequently is a history of some local injury preceding the onset, or at least the recognition, of the tumor. Such a possible association with injury is in keeping with the increased incidence of this form of cancer in boys, and in particular athletic boys, as compared to girls. The tumor forms a local painfully expanding swelling in the vicinity of a joint, and unless arrested is spread rapidly by the bloodstream, principally to the lungs. Until recently the results of treatment were abysmal. The choice lay between immediate amputation of the diseased limb on diagnosis, and radiotherapy to the tumor and delayed amputation if no metastases were apparent within six months. Intensive chemotherapeutic regimes have now been developed that can improve this dismal situation, and in certain circumstances their skilled use combined with judicious radiotherapy to the primary tumor can permit the surgical removal of the tumor without the need for amputation. Although such recent advances are encouraging, osteogenic sarcoma still remains one of the most vicious of all cancers and one of the most difficult to treat. Little evidence about the value of ascorbate therapy for this kind of cancer is as yet available.

Ewing's sarcoma is a confusing pathological entity, a comparatively rare rapidly-expanding radio-sensitive tumor of bone seen predominantly in children and young teenagers. The confusion arises because many patients so diagnosed prove in time to be suffering from a solitary bone metastasis from an unsuspected primary neuroblastoma (see below). Treatment is by local radiotherapy and systemic chemotherapy, and with modern techniques an increasing number of cures are being recorded.

A *chondroma* is a benign tumor of cartilage, often arising in childhood, which continues to grow slowly throughout adult life and may attain a great size. After many years, a high proportion of such benign tumors become malignant *chondrosarcomas*, with a brisk spurt in growth and blood-borne metastases, usually to the lungs. The peak incidence is therefore well into adult life and the common primary sites are within the thoracic cage or the pelvis. Once malignant, such tumors are virtually untreatable.

Synoviosarcomas are extremely rare malignant tumors arising from joint surfaces, usually involving the knee. They can occur at any age after childhood and they metastasize to the lungs. Standard treatment by amputation has had many failures. Current treatment trends rely more upon local radiotherapy and systemic chemotherapy, but successes are still unpredictable.

A *myoma* is a benign tumor of muscle tissue, the commonest site being in the uterus, the so-called *fibroid*, frequently multiple. Malignant tumors of muscle origin are rather rare. They arise *de novo* or more commonly by malignant change in a previously benign myoma. Such malignant muscle tumors are classified as being either *leiomyosarcomas*, if they arise from the unstriated involuntary muscles of the gastrointestinal tract, uterus, or urinary tract, etc., or the even rarer *rhabdomyosarcomas*, if they arise from the striated voluntary muscles of the musculo-skeletal system. If the tumor is anatomically accessible the treatment is by surgery; because rhabdomyosarcomas are usually highly differentiated, radiotherapy and chemotherapy have very limited value.

Fibrosarcomas are also rather rare tumors arising from the fibroblasts of connective tissue, and they exhibit all grades of behavior from the almost benign to the most malignant. They arise most commonly at sites of intense fibroblastic activity, as in old wounds, in scars, around chronic discharging sinuses, and not infrequently at the treated site many years after the over-zealous use of radiotherapy for some other form of malignancy. Their response to standard methods of treatment depends upon their anatomical site, governing the feasibility of surgical excision, and their cellular structure, governing their likely response to radiotherapy and chemotherapy.

A *lipoma* is a very common slow-growing quite benign tumor of the adipose cells, usually situated in the subcutaneous tissues. Lipomas are frequently multiple. Very rarely, a benign lipoma will undergo malignant transformation to form a *liposarcoma*. Such a transformation is heralded by a brisk spurt in growth, perhaps ulceration, and soon the appearance of widespread blood-borne metastases. The only really effective treatment is to remove all lipomas when they are still benign, even though the risk of malignant change is somewhat remote.

A *spindle-cell sarcoma* is a tumor so rapidly growing and so undifferentiated that its precise cell-type of origin cannot be determined on microscopic examination. In this respect it resembles the anaplastic carcinomas. It can arise almost anywhere in the body and it is highly malignant. By the latter token, good responses can be expected from radiotherapy and chemotherapy.

Lymphosarcomas and reticulum cell sarcomas will be discussed in the following paragraph. There are some types of sarcoma even rarer than the examples that we have discussed, such as *angiosarcomas* (arising from blood vessels), and hybrid forms such as *carcinosarcomas* and *melanosarcomas* (in which the malignancy affects both the primary cell type and the cells of the surrounding stroma), but these are little more than pathological curiosities.

CANCERS OF THE LYMPHATIC SYSTEM

The lymphatic system comprises the body-wide system of lymphatics draining into innumerable lymph nodes, and the richest source of lymphocytes of all, the spleen. This whole system is actively engaged in protection against cancer, and in passing it might be of interest to note that metastases hardly ever occur in the spleen in spite of its generous blood supply. Some constituent cells of the lymphoid system, however, may themselves become malignant. Such lymphoid malignancies may be of all grades of aggressiveness, ranging from the almost benign *follicular lymphoma* at one end of the scale, through *lymphosarcoma* and *Hodgkin's disease*, to *reticulum cell sarcoma* at the other. Because of the extensive ramifications of the lymphatic system and because of the high proliferative capacity of these lymphocyte-forming cells even under normal circumstances, such forms of malignancy, with the exception of the most benign, tend to spread widely and rapidly throughout the body, and occasionally to spill over into the bloodstream, where they are identified as either acute or chronic lymphatic leukemia (leukemia will be dealt with separately in the following section).

Benign follicular lymphoma presents itself as a painless enlargement of one lymph gland or a closely related group of lymph glands, and microscopic examination shows that the cell pattern and lymph-node architecture are still reasonably well preserved. It can be cured by simply excising the enlarged glands.

Until a comparatively short time ago, all other varieties of these lymphoid cancers were uniformly fatal in a matter of months or years, depending upon the grade of malignancy. Today, thanks to the combined use of radiotherapy and chemotherapy, a very significant proportion of patients with these diseases can be cured.

Precisely because such a high proportion of these patients can now be cured by conventional means, it would be ethically quite wrong to suggest vitamin C as an alternate form of treatment. We have, however, had limited experience with a few patients in this category who, for one reason or another, were not given adequate chemotherapy, but who were given large doses of vitamin C and who enjoyed a significant therapeutic response.

In many patients the cause of lymphatic cancers is unknown. There is a suggestion that an infectious agent may be at work, because cases tend to occur in clusters in precise geographical locations down to certain streets in certain towns, and because similar types of cancer can be produced in experimental animals by viruses. There is also a greatly increased incidence of such disorders (and the related leukemias) in people exposed to excessive high-energy radiation, such as professional radiologists and dentists, the offspring of mothers having abdominal x-rays during pregnancy, atom-bomb survivors, workers in the nuclear industry, and also patients taking immunosuppressive drugs following organ transplantation.

THE LEUKEMIAS AND OTHER
CANCERS OF THE BLOOD-FORMING CELLS

Leukemia is a form of malignancy characterized by the appearance of enormous numbers of white blood cells in the circulating blood. There are two main forms of leukemia, according to the primary cell type. These are designated *lymphatic* and *myeloid*. Lymphatic leukemia arises, as we have seen, from a primary malignancy of the lymphatic system, and the circulating blood contains an immense number of lymphocytes, whereas myeloid leukemia arises from the leukocyte-forming myeloid cells of the bone marrow and is characterized by an enormous preponderance of granulocytes in free circulation together with blast cells, which are primitive cells escaping from the marrow before maturation. Each category is further subdivided into *acute* and *chronic*, depending upon the degree of malignancy, with the acute varieties tending to be much more common in children but by no means confined to this age group.

The symptoms of leukemia are increasing lassitude, anemia, ease of bruising, susceptibility to infections, loss of weight, night sweats, splenic and often liver enlargement, and in the case of the lymphatic leukemias palpable enlargement of numerous lymph glands. The diagnosis can be established by a simple differential blood count. Not so very many years ago the leukemias were invariably fatal, in a very short time for the acute lymphatic leukemias of childhood, and in a matter of months for the chronic myeloid leukemias of adulthood. Today, thanks to major advances in chemotherapy combined with radiotherapy, an increasing number of such patients can be cured, but such successful treatment requires special expertise and often special hospital facilities.

The symptoms of acute leukemia are identical to the symptoms of scurvy, and it is well established that the circulating white cells in leukemia are abnormally low in vitamin C content. This suggests that correction of the deficit by increasing intake of vitamin C should be beneficial to the leukemic patient (see Chapters 17 on).

Polycythemia vera is a comparatively rare cancer of the bone-marrow cells responsible for red blood cell production. As a result of this disease circulating blood contains many more red blood cells than normal, leading to the characteristic florid plethoric appearance. Although malignant, the disease usually pursues a relatively benign course, with frequent survival for very many years. Some control can be achieved by regular venesection (blood-letting) and the use of radioactive isotopes such as radio-chromium, which selectively localize in bone and cause marrow suppression.

Multiple myelomatosis is a not uncommon cancer of the plasma cells of the bone marrow concerned with the production of immunoglobulins. It is more common in men than in women and tends to occur in the later decades of life. The tumor cells produce an abnormal immunoglobulin that can be detected in the blood and, in many patients, in the urine. Indeed, one possible complication of this form of cancer is kidney failure from blockage of the tubules of the kidney by this abnormal protein. The illness may run a variable course but the usual picture is one of multiple painful expanding lesions of the skull and skeleton. Treatment, if required, is by chemotherapy.

Because vitamin C in adequate amounts is needed for healthy lymphocyte production, the maturation of the red blood cells, and the production of immunoglobulins, we have been asked whether the administration of vitamin C might not aggravate rather than benefit the malignancies, lymphatic leukemia, polycythemia, and myelomatosis. The question is a serious one and the answer is not known. In our opinion aggravation by vitamin C would be highly unlikely because in each instance we are dealing with a clone of unrestrained purposeless cells. Fortunately the response to treatment can be quickly checked in all three disorders by lymphocyte count, red cell count, or measurement of the abnormal immunoglobulin, any increase indicating aggravation and any reduction indicating a beneficial response.

TUMORS OF THE BRAIN

Tumors of the brain may be benign or malignant, and because of the rigid containment of the skull they cause equal havoc by brain compression. There are two main tumor types, *meningiomas* (arising from the membranes covering the brain) and *gliomas* (arising from the brain cells). There are many varieties of the latter, such as *astrocytomas, oligodendrocytomas,* and *medulloblastomas,* classified according to primary cell type. For our purpose it is sufficient to note that all these varieties of intracranial tumors may be relatively benign, slow-growing, and well-encapsulated and, therefore, if other anatomical considerations permit, suitable for clean surgical removal with minimal damage to brain structure, or highly malignant and diffusely infiltrative with little prospect of any neurosurgical success. However, like every other form of cancer, these highly malignant tumors respond well to radiotherapy, which can offer considerable palliation and even the occasional cure. Brain tumors can occur at any age, but have a peak incidence in children up to the age of 10 and again in the fifth decade of life. Their causation has often been related to previous head injury but the evidence for this is extremely tenuous. The symptoms are increasing headache and interference with some specific brain function, depending upon the anatomical site.

CHORIOCARCINOMA

The rare tumor choriocarcinoma is unique in that it consists of cells of one individual growing and disseminating in the body of another. In every pregnancy, cells of embryonic origin form a placenta which locally invades the lining of the maternal uterus to obtain a blood supply for the developing fetus. In some rare circumstances following a normal delivery, but far more commonly after the spontaneous abortion of a grossly deformed fetus, some of these embryonic placental cells remain and assume all the characteristics of an independent highly aggressive tumor. Tumors of this sort are confined to females of child-bearing age with a recent history of pregnancy. Such a tumor can be diagnosed by a specific urine hormone test, and today is almost always curable by appropriate chemotherapy.

THE EMBRYONAL TUMORS

Embryonal tumors are a rare group of rapidly growing highly malignant tumors that afflict infants and young children and that are thought to have arisen from some slight fault in embryonic development leaving just one, or at the most a few, developing cells independent of the usual regulatory restraints. Many such tumors are already present at birth. Representative examples of such tumors are the nephroblastomas (so-called Wilms' tumors) of the kidney, retinoblastomas of the eye, medulloblastomas of the brain, neuroblastomas of the sympathetic nervous system, primitive rhabdomyosarcomas of the pelvic organs, hepatoblastomas of the liver, and a few more. All such embryonal growths are characterized by their precocious age incidence and by their tendency towards rapid growth and extreme invasiveness, although as everywhere in cancer variants can occur, with some examples exhibiting slower growth and with clinical recognition delayed until late childhood. Treatment in all such situations is extremely difficult, but combinations of radiotherapy and chemotherapy with surgical excision where possible have sometimes been successful.

THE TERATOMAS

Teratomas are tumors of varying grades of malignancy that contain an admixture of multiple tissues in various grades of differentiation. Thus a relatively benign teratoma of the ovary may contain such surprising structures as recognizable teeth, hair, skin, and miniscule bones, whereas a more malignant teratoma of, for example, the testis may consist of a solid fleshy mass which only on microscopic examination is seen to consist of individual cells of many different types. Such a bizarre appearance has led to the suggestion that a teratoma is a suppressed twin growing within the tissues of the survivor. Teratomas, however, are not confined to infancy and childhood and have a predilection for occurring in either the ovary or the testis, so that it is likely that they represent malignant degeneration arising in germ cells. Their symptoms and management depend upon anatomical site and degree of cellular differentiation.

CONCLUSION

In this chapter we have briefly summarized the usual progression of most of the common forms of cancer, with consideration in each instance of the conventional forms of treatment available and their chances of success. Again it must be mentioned that, in contrast to the space we have allotted in our discussion, the carcinomas, which are discussed in the first two-thirds of this chapter, account for over 90 percent of all human cancers and are predominantly diseases of the middle-aged and elderly. The sarcomas account for less than 5 percent of all cancers and tend to occur in much younger age groups. The other cancers can afflict any age group from infancy to old age and, although individually distinct, account for a relatively small proportion of all malignancies.

PART II
THE TREATMENT
OF CANCER

4

The Treatment of Cancer

Despite the expenditure of more than ten billion dollars on cancer research, there has been little change during the past quarter century in the mortality of most kinds of cancer. The fraction of deaths caused by cancer remains as large as before, and the amount of suffering by cancer patients may actually have increased, because some of the forms of treatment that have become popular cause the patient increased misery.

It may be that the failure of cancer research during the last decade or two has resulted from the conviction that we should strive to reach a goal that is in fact unattainable, the discovery of a miraculous "cure for cancer." This effort has diverted attention from less ambitious but potentially more profitable approaches, such as finding ways to decrease the incidence of cancer, ways of increasing the life span of the patient after he develops cancer, and ways of improving the quality of his life during the period of his survival, with the hope also that his health will be so improved as to permit him as long a life as he would have had if he had not been struck by this disease.

It is realistic to recognize that a diagnosis of cancer is often a death sentence, but not always, and not necessarily an immediate one. Some cancer patients recover completely, either because the treatment has been timely and effective or because the patient has experienced what is called a spontaneous regression. The so-called spontaneous regressions probably are in fact not really spontaneous, but rather the result of some change in the nutrition or environment of the patient that stimulates his natural protective mechanisms to such an extent as to permit them to overpower the renegade cells. But even if the disease is not overcome it may be possible to extend the time between the date of diagnosis and the date of death, and, much more important, to ensure that the person with cancer spends this intervening time not as an invalid but as an active and reasonably healthy human being. *We believe that the main objective of cancer treatment should be to give the patient a long, useful, comfortable, contented, productive, and satisfying life.*

The kinds of treatment available to achieve this desirable outcome are (a) surgery, (b) radiotherapy, (c) chemotherapy, (d) hormone therapy, (e) immunotherapy, (f) general supportive measures, (g) supplemental ascorbate (vitamin C), and (h) other nutritional or unconventional treatments, used either alone or in various combinations. It is important that the particular treatment or combination of treatments that is decided on be tailored to the needs of the individual; that is, the patient should be treated, not the disease. The comfort of the patient and his own wishes should always be considered when a decision about treatment is being made. In cancer, to a greater extent than in any other disease, the results of injudicious treatment may actually be worse than the disease itself, including needless suffering and even the shortening of life.

The values and the limitations of the different kinds of treatment of cancer are discussed in the following chapters.

The first point to note is that for many of the commoner forms of cancer the cause is already known and in some instances the cancer could be prevented and in others at least reduced. The second point to note is that for the majority of established cancers surgical excision of the growth within the limits of spread still offers the best prospects of cure, but that because of various anatomical considerations surgical removal is often technically impossible. Cancer chemotherapy is of very real value in the treatment of some leukemias and related malignancies of the lymphoid system and in the management of some other forms of malignancy characterized by very rapid growth rates, but is of very limited value elsewhere. Improvement in the scope and effectiveness of chemotherapy will undoubtedly occur, but the time scale is likely to be long and it seems probable that the vast majority of the common cancers of adulthood and old age will remain stubbornly resistant to this form of therapeutic approach. Radiotherapy is of excellent value as an adjunct to surgery in many situations, in association with chemotherapy in some others, and used alone can be quite curative in such quite different clinical problems as superficial skin cancers and deeply invasive cancers of the bladder.

While these are all very real therapeutic achievements, they are hardly grounds for complacency. It has been roughly estimated that in an average large general hospital dealing with all sorts of cancer presenting for the first time at all stages of the illness, it is possible by conventional methods to cure one third of such patients, and that another third are clearly incurable at the time of first diagnosis, leaving a middle third who might appear to be cured by the timely application of appropriate treatment, but who later relapse with untreatable recurrence of their disease and then die. A success rate of one in three is a fairly dismal record in the management of any disease, and especially in the management of a disease with such a high incidence as cancer. Often the chances of cure can be increased by early diagnosis, but even then there is no guarantee of success.

Some early and apparently very favorable patients will, in spite of adequate treatment, still die in a matter of months, whereas other apparently advanced unfavorable patients treated inadequately will confound all predictions and survive for years.

It is this baffling unpredictability of cancer progression that makes study of the whole disease so difficult. One can only talk of treatment benefits by considering trends in very large groups of patients. For reasons already mentioned, and discussed in detail in Chapter 14 and the following chapters, we are convinced that the regular ingestion of large doses of ascorbate would improve these general trends. The practical results of this policy together with some illustrative case histories of ascorbate-treated patients are given in Chapters 18 to 21.

5

The Treatment of
Cancer by Surgery

The most common initial treatment of cancer is surgery. If the tumor is still localized (Stage I, Stage II, and some Stage III), the only effective treatment is to remove it. Even if the malignant growth has already spread beyond the limits of surgical resection, removal of the main tumor may still result in cure by ridding the body of the main tumor burden, leaving the body's immune systems to mop up or constrain any malignant cells that have already escaped. Finally, even in totally incurable situations surgery may be of some value for the relief of distressing symptoms.

The type of surgery to be performed depends upon the anatomical site of the tumor, its size and the extent of local spread, and the technical problems of reconstitution and repair.

Let us consider a single example. A cancer of the lower part of the stomach is accessible, and it is easily removable unless it has infiltrated adjacent organs. Moreover, gastro-intestinal continuity can be safely restored by joining together the upper stomach remnant to a loop of small intestine. This operation, called partial gastrectomy, has virtually no mortality rate if it is done by an experienced surgeon (Figure 5-1).

The picture is completely different, however, if the tumor is situated at the upper end of the stomach. The tumor is then accessible only with difficulty, and may require a combined thoraco-abdominal incision for adequate exposure. Opening the wall of the chest adds significantly to the risk of postoperative complications. The removal of the tumor entails the removal of the whole stomach and the spleen (Figure 5-2). Most important of all, reconstitution requires the joining of the lower esophagus to the jejunum (a part of the small intestine), and even in the most experienced hands such a junction may

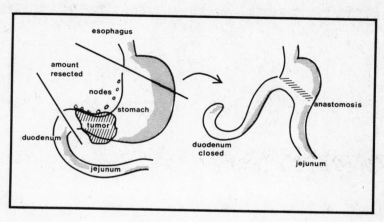

FIGURE 5-1
Partial gastrectomy for cancer of low stomach.

leak, with disastrous consequences for the patient in the immediate post-operative period. This operation, which is called total gastrectomy, carries an appreciably greater risk than partial gastrectomy. Thus the degree of success of an operation is determined in part by the anatomical site of the tumor.

The type of surgery that should be performed is also limited by the general condition of the patient and by the evidence about the extent to which the cancer has spread. Thus a partial gastrectomy might be justified in a frail elderly patient with cardio-respiratory problems because of the low operative risks involved, whereas a total gastrectomy under such circumstances would be very unwise, with a high probability of abruptly shortening the patient's life. Similarly, in the presence of metastases in the liver a partial gastrectomy is still often justifiable for the sake of symptomatic relief, increasing the comfort of the patient during the remainder of his life, whereas a total gastrectomy in such an incurable situation would most certainly not be justifiable.

The really significant improvements in the treatment of cancer during the last thirty years have come from advances in surgery, the development of new techniques, and especially from improved methods of anesthesia, the availability of antibiotics to control post-operative infections, better blood-transfusion services, and a better understanding and practice of procedures of intensive care. These broad advances have enabled surgeons to undertake with confidence extensive resections in Stage-III cancer patients that could not have been contemplated a quarter of a century ago. By enabling more and more such patients to survive the immediate post-operative period after cancer

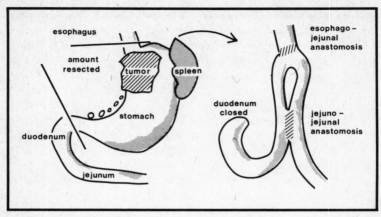

FIGURE 5-2
Total gastrectomy for cancer of high stomach.

resection, they give a better chance of long-term survival. It is ironic that the significant improvements in cancer survival compared to thirty years ago owe very little to research on cancer itself.

Bigger surgery, however, does not always mean better surgery, and a technical triumph for the surgeon and his team may be a disaster for the patient. Evaluating the real worth of an extensive operating procedure should be based on the subsequent quality of life of the patient rather than just on the prolongation of his survival. Thus it is technically possible to remove the whole pancreas in a patient with pancreatic cancer, but the operation carries such a high immediate post-operative mortality and leaves the surviving patients in such a state of chronic invalidism that few surgeons would now advise it.

Even with the situation of cancer of the upper stomach discussed above, the surgeon faces deep ethical problems. A surgeon of good average experience and competence might operate on ten of these patients, and it would really be no reflection on his technical ability if two died within the first week from severe post-operative complications. Of the remaining eight, seven might die of recurrence of their cancer within a year, leaving one patient potentially cured. Most surgeons would take the view that all ten patients were going to die anyway, and to have even one long-term survivor should be regarded as a gain. It is a very difficult moral question to decide whether surgically killing two patients and making another seven go through all the major trauma and post-operative morbidity of major surgery that was useless to them is outbalanced by the real gain of one patient. We believe that most informed patients would be willing to take the chance of 1 in 10 of being the fortunate long-term survivor, but would prefer to have a treatment involving a smaller immediate risk and a smaller amount of suffering and giving a roughly equal chance of long-term survival, if such a treatment were available.

The fact that bigger surgery is not necessarily better surgery is well illustrated by the current dilemma facing surgeons in the treatment of the most common of all cancers among women, cancer of the breast. For many years the standard treatment has been the operation of radical mastectomy that was pioneered by William Halsted of Johns Hopkins Hospital, Baltimore, around the turn of the century. The operation as originally devised consisted of removing the entire breast with a large circle of skin overlying the tumor, removing the two underlying main chest-wall muscles leading to the shoulder, with careful dissection of these structures from the ribcage, and the careful and meticulous surgical dissection and removal of all the lymph nodes in the axilla (armpit). This was an extensive and very mutilating procedure, leaving the woman not only without a breast but also with a deep depression where the underlying muscles had been removed, an ugly scar, and almost always a permanent brawny swelling of the arm because of the surgical interference with its lymphatic drainage. Nevertheless the operation soon became established all over the world because it satisfied the basic surgical principle of removing the main tumor and its related lymph drainage and because a large number of women who had had the operation survived for many years and seemed to have been cured.

Over the years, the operation was slightly modified by the removal of less skin and sometimes less muscle, but the basic extent of the resection remained much the same.

Then just after the Second World War there came the news from Scotland that simple mastectomy (removing the diseased breast only and leaving the axillary contents and underlying muscles undisturbed), followed by carefully planned radiotherapy to the chest wall and axilla, produced results that were not just as good but in fact were somewhat better than those of the radical procedure. (By "results" is meant the fraction of patients still alive five years after the diagnosis of breast cancer.) For a time American and British surgery parted ways, with American surgeons relying on the well-established and tested Halsted procedure and British surgeons adopting the much less mutilating simple mastectomy plus radiotherapy.

Then, around the early 1950s, two further developments occurred that were even more divergent. On the basis of the advances in techniques of anesthesia and resuscitation mentioned earlier the operation called super-radical mastectomy was developed in the United States. This operation consists of the standard·Halsted procedure extended by surgically removing all the lymph nodes on that side of the neck, opening the thoracic cage, and dissecting out all the lymph nodes along the internal mammary chain beneath the breastbone and in front of the heart. This operation seemed to be justified by the fact that in a significant fraction of the patients these deeply concealed lymph glands were found to be already invaded by the malignant cells. However, although such extensive surgery appeared to be based on sound principles, the results of the procedure showed no advantage over those for less radical procedures, and super-radical mastectomy has few proponents today.

Also in the early fifties, there came a report from Finland that simply to remove the tumor without removing the whole breast (called lumpectomy or tylectomy) offered not just as good but in fact somewhat better prospects of survival than mastectomy. The Finnish claim has been the subject of a controlled trial in London during recent years, in which patients with their informed consent are randomly allocated to one group treated by simple mastectomy or to another group treated by lumpectomy. The results so far indicate that the patients treated by lumpectomy are doing marginally better than those treated by mastectomy.

Here we have two widely divergent procedures: an extremely radical operation to remove all malignant tissues, and the simple removal of the obvious lump, with the claim that the patients who are given this simple surgical treatment do just as well as those who suffer the trauma of the extensive surgery. Moreover, the Edinburgh surgeons who introduced simple mastectomy plus radiotherapy have recently reported that the patients who receive simple mastectomy alone do marginally better than those who also are given radiotherapy.

The observations from Halsted on seem to be showing that the less that is done for breast-cancer patients, the better their chances of survival. The damage done to the body by surgical or radiotherapeutic intervention may be greater than the benefit resulting from partial control of the disease. This trend has led many thoughtful surgeons to question seriously whether they should treat breast-cancer patients at all—whether these patients might not better be left alone. The question is a serious one, demanding an answer.

A significant step forward was made in 1956 by Hardin B. Jones. He pointed out that much of the statistical information about the average times of survival of cancer patients given different treatments is unreliable because of uncertainty about the date from which survival is measured. Cancer differs from other diseases in a remarkable way. With most diseases it is found that almost all the patients live for about the same length of time after diagnosis and then either die or recover. With patients who have been diagnosed as having a certain kind of cancer, however, or have reached a certain stage in the disease the death rate is nearly constant: the same fraction of the survivors in the group die each day, day after day. He stated that, with few exceptions, "Groups with cancer maintain the same death rate throughout the disease, and the death rate does not advance with duration of the disease." Accordingly, he said, the best way of comparing two alternative treatments of patients with the same kind of cancer is to observe the death rates of groups treated in the two ways. He applied this way of analyzing the survival curves to the reported observations on patients with different kinds of cancer, including breast cancer, and he reached the conclusion that survival of patients with breast cancer is not changed very much by treatment. Patients treated by radical mastectomy have the same death rate after the operation as those treated by simple mastectomy, and even the same as those who received no treatment.

A recent study of the problem of the treatment of breast cancer has been published by McPherson and Fox (1977). They mention that breast cancer is one of the major causes of death in women, especially in the United States and Europe, that in the United States there are about 90,000 new cases per year, and that about 7,000,000 U.S. women now alive will have this disease sometime in their lifetime. After mentioning the work of Hardin Jones and making a careful analysis of the results of eight recent clinical trials, they reached the following conclusions:

1. Radical mastectomy (with radiotherapy) is equivalent in terms of survival experience to simple mastectomy plus postoperative radiotherapy. In terms of mutilation, morbidity, length of convalescence, and time taken for the wound to heal, the differences are substantial.

2. For patients without clinical evidence of involved nodes, local removal of the tumor (tylectomy) plus radiotherapy appears to be equivalent in terms of survival experience to radical mastectomy (except for a somewhat higher incidence of local recurrence).

3. Postoperative radiotherapy seems, however, to offer little benefit and may be detrimental for some patients.

McPherson and Fox point out that in the United States radical mastectomy is the treatment given to some 80 percent of patients with breast cancer, showing that these conclusions are not widely agreed upon, and say that "If there were one randomized series which showed a significant advantage in terms of 'cure' rate or length of survival, then presumably the radical operation could be justified on some evaluation of quantity of life against quality. However, there appears to be no such evidence."

To explain the far greater use of radical mastectomy in the United States than in Europe they mention as the first reason the great reputation of Halsted and of the Johns Hopkins School of Medicine at the beginning of the 20th Century, and then say

> The second reason invokes the possible influence of fee-for-service medicine on conditioning behavior. In short, when the fee schedules for radical mastectomy are sometimes more than twice as high as those for simple mastectomy, it would be difficult to argue that this would have no effect on the decisions of some physicians, particularly where there is little evidence that simple mastectomy and radiotherapy constitute a more effective treatment. . . . Moreover, the escalating risk of malpractice litigation in the event of a recurrence of the disease is likely to have the effect of encouraging as much intervention as possible. . . .

We may ask why there is little difference in survival of patients who are treated by simple mastectomy and those who receive an extended operation, with removal of lymph nodes, which often contain malignant cells. The answer may be that the lymph nodes are part of our system of protective mechanisms, which if undisturbed may be able to overcome the malignancy, but which is significantly damaged by removal of the nodes.

The same conclusion has been reached from the study of patients with cancer of the colon. Warren Cole and his associates in Chicago developed a method of detecting cancer cells in the peripheral blood, presumably on the way to form metastases. They found that during surgical resection of a colonic cancer a sample of blood drawn from a vein in the arm quite frequently, but not always, contained clumps of cancer cells. At follow-up studies after five years they found no significant difference in survival times between those patients who had had detectable cancer cells floating in their blood and those who had not, whereas it would be expected that those patients with cancer cells in their circulation would have a much greater incidence of metastases.

The conclusion is that the natural protective mechanisms of the human body are usually able to restrain and to destroy these residual cancer cells. The importance of these natural protective mechanisms can hardly be overemphasized. The relation between surgery, as well as other treatments, and the natural protective mechanisms needs to be examined with care. We shall return to this subject in later chapters.

Surgical intervention is effective, at least at some stages, against cancer of the breast, stomach, small and large intestines, bladder, uterus, kidney, testis, ovary, brain, bone, and muscle. While surgery, if possible, must always remain the first line of treatment for cancer, a rather conservative approach may often be justified. There are probably few indications now, except for the relief of particularly distressing symptoms, for the type of very extensive anatomical dissections that modern techniques of anesthesia and resuscitation have made possible.

For many cancer patients surgery is the best primary treatment. There is no incompatibility between surgery and an increased intake of vitamin C, as discussed later in this book.

6

The Treatment of Cancer by Radiotherapy

X-rays were discovered by the German physicist Wilhelm Konrad Röntgen in 1895 and radioactivity was discovered in 1896 by the French physicist Henri Becquerel, who showed that compounds of uranium emit a kind of radiation, called gamma rays, resembling x-rays. It was soon recognized that both x-rays and gamma rays damage tissues and can cause cancer. It was also discovered that these rays damage malignant tissues more than normal tissues, and this discovery soon led to their use in the treatment of cancer. In those early days, results that seemed almost miraculous were obtained. Thus a squamous epithelioma of the lip, a nasty raised unsightly ulcerated tumor that would have required fairly extensive and cosmetically disfiguring surgery for its removal, could be exposed to x-rays or to radioactivity (by the implanatation of a hollow needle containing radium or radon), and within a few weeks the tumor would have disappeared, leaving only a small scar. This was a very significant therapeutic achievement.

X-rays are electromagnetic waves, similar to infrared, visible, and ultraviolet light and to radio waves. They are produced in an x-ray tube. Electrons are boiled out of a hot wire, which serves as the cathode, and are accelerated by the applied electric potential difference (voltage) toward the anode, a metal plate. When an electron strikes the anode and is brought to a sudden stop its kinetic energy is converted into an x-ray quantum, a photon. With a potential difference of 50,000 to 1 million volts, each of these x-ray photons has energy between 6,000 and 120,000 times that of a photon in the near ultraviolet part of sunlight (3.3 volts), which itself can damage tissues, causing sunburn and skin cancer. X-rays and gamma rays, as well as certain other rays, are called *high-energy radiation*.

The gamma rays from a radioactive isotope of cobalt, cobalt 60, which is produced in a nuclear reactor, are also used in cancer therapy. A small amount of cobalt 60 is placed in a container with thick lead walls and a small hole through which a beam of gamma rays can escape. These gamma rays are essentially the same as million-volt x-rays.

For reasons to be discussed later, not all tumors respond to x-rays or gamma rays. In an attempt to overcome this problem, scientists are beginning to study the effects of other high-energy rays or particles on cancer. Fast neutrons, protons, pions, and other projectiles are being tested. These applications of high-energy physics to cancer offer some promise, but at the present time they are in the experimental stage.

Although these high-energy rays differ somewhat from one another, their effect on the tissues is about the same, and for simplicity we may talk about radiation (meaing high-energy radiation). The effect of radiation on tissues is mainly *to damage and destroy dividing cells*. There is also another effect, which may be almost as important in the treatment of cancer. This is *to damage the ground substance* (the intercellular cement) of the whole field that is irradiated, leaving a scarred and much more resistant local environment for the tumor cells that have survived the initial assault.

Because many tumor cells are dividing at a higher rate than the cells of the normal tissues, the radiation inflicts more damage on the tumor than on the normal tissues. Also, the more rapidly proliferating, the more anaplastic (primitive, embryonic), and the more undifferentiated the tumor, the more likely will it be to respond to radiation. It seems paradoxical that it is the most malignant tumors that respond best to treatment with high-energy radiation. The same paradox applies also to cytotoxic chemotherapy. Slowly growing tumors respond poorly to radiotherapy; they are said to be radiation-resistant. To inflict sufficient radiation damage on such a tumor would result in intolerable damage to the normal tissues.

One way out of this difficulty is to irradiate through multiple portals of entry; that is, if the directions of the beams are carefully calculated and adjusted, it is possible to deliver a high dose of radiation to the tumor while subjecting the skin and intervening tissues to only a tolerable dose.

Radiotherapy may be employed in certain situations as the only form of treatment, or as an adjunct to surgery, given either pre-operatively, to shrink the main tumor and to limit the spreading tendency of peripheral cells, or post-operatively, to mop up any tumor cells left behind at surgery, or it may be used in combination with chemotherapeutic regimes. It may be radical, with use of high doses in the hope of effecting a cure, or palliative, with use of smaller doses given to achieve some symptomatic relief. An example of the former is the use of large amounts of megavoltage (million volt) radiation through multiple portals for the cure of cancer of the bladder, and an example of the latter is a single accurately directed exposure to relieve the pain of a skeletal metastasis.

Radiation treatment may also be given internally by implanting a radioactive source in or near the tumor. An example already mentioned is that of implanting a radium needle (a hollow stainless steel receptacle for the radioactive substance) for treatment of cancer of the lip or tongue. Intra-cavitary radium therapy is also successful in the cure of cancer of the cervix, one of the common forms of cancer in women; the results obtained by competent use of radiotherapy are as good as those by fairly extensive surgery.

In a few situations the benefits of radiation therapy can be achieved by using isotopes that localize within the tumor. Thyroid tissue concentrates iodine from the blood, and some thyroid cancers retain this ability. Thus by first stimulating such cells to high activity by giving thyroid-stimulating hormone and then having the patient drink a solution containing a radioactive isotope of iodine much of the radioactivity will be concentrated in the various deposits of the tumor, and the high-energy rays will have the highly specific effect of destroying only the tumor cells. Another example of this technique is the use of a radioactive isotope of phosphorous, which concentrates in the bones and selectively irradiates tumors of bone and bone marrow.

Damage to the skin with external irradiation is usually limited to mild erythema (redness) at the point of entry, with later dry scaling and mild pigmentation. If, however, too high doses are used or the patient is unusually sensitive a true radiation burn may result, leading in severe instances to complete destruction of the skin. High doses also may lead to radiation-necrosis (destruction) of bone, which can be a very troublesome complication of injudicious radiation therapy. Fortunately these complications are extremely rare. But some complications have to be accepted, when weighed against the long-term gain from the treatment. Thus in treating cancer of the bladder with megavoltage external irradiation (usually considered to be the only alternative to removal of the bladder and transplantation of the ureters into the colon) it is just not possible to avoid irradiating the normal rectum. Thus diarrhea from damage to the rectal mucosa is an almost invariable accompaniment of radiotherapy of cancer of the bladder; but eventually the rectal mucosa will recover, the diarrhea will cease, and the patient may be cured.

The general side-effects of radiation therapy depend upon the volume of the tissue that is irradiated. They will be completely absent in, for example, treatment of a small cancer of the lip, but may be quite disabling in radiation treatment of cancer of the breast, where we are also forced to expose to radiation the underlying lung and rib cage, right through to the shoulder blade. These side effects comprise feelings of lassitude and very often nausea, sometimes proceeding to vomiting; they gradually disappear when the course of radiotherapy is terminated. If the field to be irradiated covers a substantial fraction of the active bone marrow—the pelvis, spine, and rib cage in adults —a marked drop in the number of circulating white cells and platelets can occur, with risk of increased susceptibility to infections and hemorrhages.

There are certain situations where these risks have to be accepted, and are acceptable provided that careful blood counts are regularly done. Among these situations are the radiation treatment of some highly radiation-sensitive brain tumors, especially in children, and the irradiation of large volumes of tissues as may be required for the control of Hodgkin's disease or of some forms of leukemia. Indeed, in certain forms of leukemia irradiation of the whole body is sometimes carried out, but in limited doses given at spaced intervals to allow the normal tissues adequate time for repair.

We conclude that high-energy radiation therapy is the second most valuable member of our conventional therapeutic armory. Used alone it can cure a variety of tumors, and used as an adjunct to surgery or to chemotherapy it can improve the chances of cure for many more. The side effects are rarely overwhelmingly severe and can be controlled by competent doctoring. It is true that some common tumors, such as cancers of the stomach and colon, are virtually unaffected by radiotherapy, but this fact serves to emphasize its value in the treatment of cancer at many other sites.

7

The Treatment of Cancer by Chemotherapy

The ideal chemotherapeutic agent for cancer would be some compound that selectively destroys every malignant cell but is completely harmless to all normal cells. In the worldwide search for such a compound, current thinking is understandably influenced by the spectacular successes of antibacterial chemotherapy. Taking the sulfonamides and penicillin as examples, we have substances that exploit explicit metabolic differences between bacterial and mammalian cells, and as a result are fatal to many bacteria in minute concentrations and harmless to the human in massive concentrations, apart from the few rare individuals who develop sensitivity reactions.

As more and more powerful antibacterial agents are discovered, synthesized, tested, and brought into successful clinical use, the trend seems to confirm the prediction made at the beginning of this century by the brilliant German chemist Paul Ehrlich, that for every disease a specific chemical compound, a "Silver Bullet," could be concocted to eradicate that disease. By patient synthesis and testing, Ehrlich developed arsphenamine, the first known specific chemical cure for a disease, the disease syphilis. In the 1930s another brilliant German chemist, Gerhard Domagk, working in the synthetic dyestuffs industry, selected one such dyestuff, prontosil rubrum, from many thousands tested, showed that it protected experimental mice from pneumonia, and gave the world the sulfonamides. During the Second World War the urgent need to protect battle casualties from gas-gangrene infection of wounds, which had been a major complication of the First World War, recalled the chance discovery of penicillin by the Scottish bacteriologist Alexander Fleming, years before. The brilliant work of Howard W. Florey and Ernst

Boris Chain then demonstrated to the world the value of this important antibiotic substance, which is effective against gas gangrene and a multitude of other infections. After this promising lead, streptomycin was soon discovered, leading to greatly increased control of tuberculosis. In the same period the tetracyclines and chloramphenicols were developed, with perhaps even greater practical impact upon the control of potentially fatal human bacterial diseases. Continuing work along these lines in many university departments and the research laboratories of the major international pharmaceutical companies has led to the discovery of so many new antibiotics and chemotherapeutic agents that it is reasonable to assume that eventually every bacterial infestation that besets mankind will be controlled and eradicated by the chemical ingenuity of mankind. These therapeutic advances deserve the highest praise.

All of this progress is based upon the exploitation of some inherent metabolic difference between the bacterial foreign-invader cells and the cells of the susceptible human victim. In our opinion, the very successes of antibacterial chemotherapy are responsible for much confusion in cancer chemotherapy research. Fundamentally, cancer cells are not foreign invaders. The malignant cells of John Doe's stomach cancer have more resemblance to the normal cells of John Doe's stomach than to any other cell in his body. These cancer cells erupting in John Doe belong to John Doe, and are fundamentally quite different from any cells, normal or malignant, present in his sister, his parents, his grandparents, or any other person, except an identical twin. Thus the basic assumption that cancer cells, like bacteria, have some fundamental difference in origin and metabolism from the cells of the host, capable of chemotherapeutic exploitation, seems to be wrong.

Progress in cancer chemotherapy was first based on the assumption that cancer cells divide at a greater rate than normal cells. Thus it was argued that any chemical poison that would preferentially destroy dividing cells would have a greater deterrent effect upon cancer cells than on the allegedly quiescent cells of the host. Almost every chemotherapeutic compound so far discovered acts in this non-specific manner, by interfering with the processes of cell division and multiplication. Comparatively recent studies on tumor-cell kinetics, however, indicate that for the majority of human cancers the cell-division rate is in fact lower than that for a wide variety of normal tissues of the host, such as skin, the lining of the gastrointestinal tract, and the bone marrow responsible for the production of the red and white blood cells and platelets.

With a better understanding, we now see that the use of cytotoxic (cell-killing) cancer chemotherapeutic agents can still be justified in such situations because of the greater recovery potential of the normal cells. The evolution of this understanding will be summarized later in this chapter, but it has to be emphasized that cancer chemotherapy owes as much to chance observation and serendipity as to exact science.

The chemical compound bis(2-chloroethyl)sulfide, $(ClCH_2CH_2)_2S$, commonly called mustard gas, is a deadly vesicant (blistering agent) that can burn the skin, the lining of the gut, with profuse and fatal vomiting and diarrhea, and the linings of the lungs, with a suffocating outpouring of fluid, and that can cause blindness. It was used extensively as a poison gas in World War I, and at that time it was observed that the survivors of a mustard-gas attack showed a sharp decrease in the number of their circulating white blood cells (a leukopenia, deficiency of leukocytes). A similar observation was made in 1944 when a U.S. military transport loaded with drums of mustard gas was sunk by enemy action in the harbor of Naples, with much loss of life. It was then recognized that this substance might have some value in the management of leukemia, a group of cancerous disorders of the blood-forming tissues that usually lead to the infusion into the circulation of enormous numbers of leukocytes. Cautious clinical trials in leukemia patients were then undertaken with nitrogen mustard, a closely related compound with chemical formula $(ClCH_2CH_2)_2NCH_3HCl$. Although no permanent cures resulted, some remissions of this otherwise fatal illness were recorded. At about the same time, the late 1940s, Sidney Farber reported the induction of somewhat similar real but transient remissions in leukemia patients by use of another drug, methotrexate, a substance similar to one of the B vitamins, folic acid, which is required for cell division. This was the exciting dawn of cancer chemotherapy, the discovery and use of the first drugs other than hormones that could significantly retard the progress of a malignant disease. With such an encouraging start, the successful chemotherapy of all cancers seemed to be just over the horizon.

As was mentioned at the start of this chapter, the ideal treatment of cancer would be one that would select and destroy the malignant cells while leaving the normal cells unharmed. Nitrogen mustard and methotrexate failed on both counts. The leukemias returned after a period of remission, and the drugs poisoned the patients, causing extremely severe side effects. Nevertheless they are somewhat more poisonous to the malignant cells than to the normal cells, so that there is some net gain.

It was then thought, and continues to be said by some investigators, that all that is needed to produce the ideal anti-cancer drug is to refine the chemotherapeutic agents somewhat. This idea is unlikely to turn out to be true, because these agents are in no way specific anti-cancer drugs.

The problem of finding a truly effective drug to control cancer is made very difficult by the fact that in any person the cancer cells are almost identical with the normal cells; they differ only in a few characteristics, which are just those needed to confer malignancy on them. A good anti-cancer drug might be one that attacked or inhibited one of these characteristics, and since a malignancy seems to involve several characteristics, it is not surprising that during recent years the oncologists have been relying on the use of two or more anti-cancer drugs, either together or in succession, rather than on a single one.

One difference in cell properties that is exploitable is that in rate of cell division. A cytotoxic (cell-poisoning) agent that would interfere with cell division would have more effect on the rapidly dividing cells of a malignant tumor than on the more slowly dividing cells of most normal tissues. Thus, as also in the case of radiotherapy, it is paradoxical but true that the more malignant, the more anaplastic, the more invasive, the more aggressive, and the more rapidly dividing the tumor, the more likely it is to respond to cytotoxic chemotherapy. The most striking successes of anticancer chemotherapy have been in rather disastrous forms of malignancy, such as the acute leukemias of childhood, Burkitt's lymphoma of equatorial Africa, and choriocarcinoma.

Among the normal tissues in which the rate of cell division is quite high are the bone marrow, which constantly produces new red blood cells, platelets, and granulocytes, the lymphoreticular system, which constantly produces new lymphocytes, the cells lining the gastrointestinal tract, and the cells of the skin and hair follicles. It is accordingly not surprising that among the side effects of the cytotoxic drugs are anemia, damage to the immune mechanisms, gastrointestinal upsets, and loss of hair.

The difference between a malignant growth and normal tissue is not the rate of cell division, but rather its control. The normal cells may be dividing rapidly, but they divide only to the extent necessary for the proper functioning of the organism. The cells of a malignant tumor are largely out of control. Some tumor cells are continually being destroyed, but the tumor may produce new ones at a far greater rate, and hence it may grow rapidly. Even a slow-growing tumor, producing new cells at only a slightly greater rate than that at which old cells are being destroyed, will still, in the course of time, cause the death of the patient.

Can cytotoxic agents be of any value in this situation? This is a hard question to answer, and many experienced clinicians have expressed their doubts.

Let us consider a fairly typical situation in "solid" cancer, where the tumor cells are proliferating at a lower rate than the cells of the bone marrow, gastro-intestinal tract, or even skin. And let us say that we decide to treat that patient by the *continuous* administration of a cytotoxic agent. This drug will kill any dividing cell, whether it be "normal" or "malignant." The treatment will certainly retard the growth of the tumor, and, because of the continuing cell loss, it may even cause it to diminish significantly in size. The destructive effects of such treatment on the more rapidly dividing normal cells will, however, be much greater. The bone marrow will be steadily damaged and will stop producing platelets, with the result that the patient may die of hemorrhage. It will stop producing granulocytes, so that the patient becomes extremely susceptible to any infection, also likely to be fatal. In time, the patient will become anemic because of the cessation of production of red blood cells. The effects on the gastro-intestinal tract will be equally disastrous. Pronounced nausea and soon vomiting will be an early sign, leading on to atrophy of the intestinal villi, constant diarrhea, and an inability to absorb any nutrient. In the skin, total hair loss will be an early feature, followed by an exfoliative dermatitis. There could be other destructive effects on normal tissues, anything from hemorrhagic cystitis to brain damage. It is clear that if we go on like this, we shall kill the patient long before we can kill the tumor. This has happened, and the tragedy is that it is still happening by the aggressive and injudicious use of cytotoxic chemotherapy.

One way out of this difficulty is to administer the cytotoxic agent on an *intermittent* basis, allowing a treatment-free interval between courses for recovery. This "pulsed-dose technique" exploits the higher proliferative capacity of the normal cells and their greater potential for recovery. The first dose is administered and all vulnerable cells, normal or malignant, are damaged, and the patient suffers most if not all the unpleasant side-effects noted above. However, during the treatment-free interval these unpleasant symptoms subside, and the bone-marrow, gastrointestinal tract, and skin recover more quickly than the tumor. If we are very clever in our measurement of the dose of the cytotoxic agent we use, and, even more important, in our decision about the length of the treatment-free interval to permit normal tissue recovery, but always keeping ahead of the tumor, it should be possible to create a situation such that we take the patient through repeated cycles of profound tissue damage but eventual repair, against a background of progressive tumor damage to the point of total eradication of the tumor. The truth is, however, that we are rarely clever enough to succeed, because we lack the means to calculate the precise dosages and timing for each individual patient. Empirical regimes have to be used, and although they meet with some success, more often we finish up either killing the patient or making him thoroughly miserable with no appreciable effect on the tumor.

And there are other difficulties. Even though we have hit upon the perfect combination and all trace of the tumor completely disappears, there could be millions of tumor cells still in existence and ready to surge into renewed activity as soon as the treatment is discontinued, and these regimes cannot be continued indefinitely. Furthermore, it is believed that the immune systems of the body play an important role in destroying tumor cells, and the immune systems are extremely vulnerable to cytotoxic agents, so what we gain in one way, we destroy in another.

Many different cytotoxic agents are now in common use, and it has been found that they are often synergistic; that is, the effect of giving two such drugs together is greater than a simple additive effect might have predicted. This is because these agents act on different phases of the cell division cycle. It is now common practice to employ multiple chemotherapy, the giving of two or more different cytotoxic agents simultaneously. An example is "MOPP" (an acronym from the active agents), introduced by the National Cancer Institute in the early sixties:

Nitrogen mustard ("Mustine") intravenously on Day 1 and Day 8

Vincristine ("Oncovin") intravenously on Day 1 and Day 8

Procarbazine ("Natulan") by mouth, daily on Days 1 to 14 inclusive

Prednisone by mouth, daily on Days 1 to 14 inclusive, during 1st and 4th courses

Six courses are given, with two weeks free of all medication between the end of one course and the beginning of the next.

This regime has proved to be particularly useful, producing a high rate of sustained remissions, in the management of Hodgkin's disease, a not uncommon malignancy of the lymphoreticular system.

For reasons not very clearly understood, clinical experience indicates that some cytotoxic agents are more effective against some types of cancer than against others, and, equally puzzling, are more toxic to one normal tissue than to another.

The drugs used against cancer may be conveniently grouped into several classes. Mustard gas and nitrogen mustard, mentioned above, are in the class of *alkylating agents*. They have the power of attaching themselves or transferring an alkyl group (such as the methyl group, $-CH_3$) to other molecules, in particular to the units (adenine, thymine, guanine, cytosine) in the DNA of the cells, and in this way interfering with cell division. The *antimetabolites* are substances closely similar to some substance that is necessary for growth and reproduction, such as a vitamin. An antimetabolite works by combining with an enzyme or other protein in the same way as does the vitamin or other important molecule, and then not carrying out the vital function, while blocking the vitamin from access; an example is methotrexate, which blocks folic acid, an important vitamin. The *mitotic inhibitors* prevent mitosis, the process in which the chromosomes in the cell duplicate themselves and then the pairs separate, in order that one set may remain in each of the two daughter cells that are formed when the cell divides. The antibiotics used in the treatment of cancer may function as mitotic inhibitors. There are also some anti-cancer drugs that have not been assigned to these classes. Some information about many of the anti-cancer drugs, especially those most used, is given in Appendix II. These drugs are all extremely potent poisons, and must be used with very great care and judgment. In the very acute anaplastic tumors and in tumors with a very high growth rate and negligible cell loss they can be remarkably effective, and through their use we can now talk of "cures" in the acute leukemias of childhood and Hodgkin's disease, a statement that would have been unthinkable even 15 years ago. Unfortunately these very responsive tumor situations are only a small minority of the broad spectrum of human cancer, less than 5 percent of all malignant disease.

The question arises as to whether cytotoxic chemotherapy has any value in the remaining 95 percent of cancer patients. Many patients doubt it, and there are sound reasons for this view. First, the side effects of cytotoxic chemotherapy can make these patients profoundly miserable, providing a situation where the treatment may be worse than the disease. And even in the best hands, the success rate is only about one in five. One patient might receive some benefit while the other four have been rendered thoroughly miserable to no advantage. And even the one success is usually comparatively short lived, frequently no more than a matter of months in the usual solid cancers of adulthood and advancing years. The tumor may shrink, and in the very successful response even apparently disappear, but it will almost invariably recur, and all that will have been gained may be a few short months at the expense of a great deal of unpleasantness and misery.

In his book *Strike Back at Cancer* Stephen A. Rapaport states that

> In sum, chemotherapy is a cancer treatment that has produced some isolated successes in certain areas but remains, on balance, an approach that is largely in its experimental stage. The cancers that have proved most responsive to chemotherapy are leukemia, cancer of the head and neck, and Hodgkin's disease, although it would be misleading to say that there are chemical 'cures' for these cancers. Probably the most important thing to bear in mind if you or someone you know is given the choice of undergoing chemotherapy is that the treatment is highly unpredictable and that the psychological make-up and tolerance level of the patient are as much a factor in the success or failure of the therapy as the therapy itself.

This may be an overpessimistic view. However, we are still faced with the question as to how to treat patients with the great majority of cancers, the solid slow-growing tumors in adults, remembering that the aim is not usually to seek an elusive "cure" but rather to extend the remaining time of life as long as possible and to ensure that the period of survival is spent in comfort, dignity, and the best possible well-being. If the tumor is still localized and its surgical removal is feasible, surgery is almost always the treatment to be chosen. If the tumor is still largely localized but has spread outside the surgical field local radiotherapy, with or without surgery, is the treatment of choice. If the tumor is widely disseminated the only conventional treatment may be chemotherapy. Whether it is used or not is a matter for the informed patient and a responsible doctor to decide, on the basis of likely response (see Chapter 23). A trial course may be justified, with further treatment determined by the nature of the response. The possible cost of the treatment also needs some consideration; to subject the patient and his family to a treatment that has little promise of success and that costs them thousands or tens of thousands of dollars may only increase the burden of their suffering. What is near-criminal is treating for treatment's sake, and both patients and many doctors may share the responsibility for such an action. Patients beg for treatment, and doctors feel an obligation to provide it, even though it may be obvious that the treatment does more harm than good. It should be kept in mind, when a decision is being made, that the natural protective mechanisms of the body, when they are given the opportunity to function most effectively, may retard and just very occasionally overcome the disease. A great disadvantage of chemotherapy is that the chemotherapeutic agents seriously damage the body's natural protective mechanisms.

8

The Treatment of
Cancer by Hormones

Hormones are substances that are secreted by cells in one part of the body, are transported by the body fluids to another part, and there produce a specific effect on the activity of cells remote from those that liberated them. Thus hormones are normal constituents of the human body, which may be described as chemical messengers; they function in the control of metabolic processes. The use of hormones in the treatment of cancer is an example of *orthomolecular* medicine, which is defined as the preservation of good health and the treatment of disease by varying the concentrations in the human body of substances that are normally present in the body and are required for health (see Chapter 14).

Some of the hormones used as anticancer agents, such as cortisone, hydrocortisone, ACTH (adrenocorticotrophic hormone), testosterone, and progesterone, are true hormones, and hence can be classed as orthomolecular substances. Others, however, are not true hormones, but are related substances that have hormonal activity or that interfere with the action of hormones, and hence are drugs rather than orthomolecular substances. Some examples are prednisone, prednisolone, fluoxymesterone, diethylstilbestrol (DES), and ethinylestradiol.

The female breast is a typical target organ under hormonal control. During the earlier part of the menstrual cycle a build-up of the female hormone (estrogen) induces the glandular cells of the breast (those from which breast cancers arise) to proliferate, but if pregnancy does not occur a different combination of hormones at the time of menstruation allows these proliferative changes to regress to be ready for the next cycle. The clock for all this regular activity is situated in the pituitary gland. If pregnancy does occur the proliferative changes continue, and at the time of birth of the infant yet another hormonal combination induces lactation. This information, at least in its rough outline, has been known for very many years.

In 1897 a surgeon in Glasgow, Scotland, Sir George Beatson, surgically removed the ovaries (the main, but not the only source of estrogen in premenopausal women) from three patients with advanced breast cancer, and noted remarkable remission of the disease in two of them.

In the 1930s and 1940s, Charles Huggins, working in Chicago, noting that the male prostate gland (a common site of cancer) is under the control of the male sex hormone secreted by the testes, produced regression in a high proportion of prostatic cancers by surgical castration, and later by "medical castration," accomplished by giving female sex hormones to the patients. Because prostatic cancer was then almost untreatable otherwise, except by very radical and debilitating surgery, this was a very significant therapeutic advance.

Thus we had two clear examples that by either removing the source of, or medically suppressing, a particular hormone, we can induce regression of cancer in the target organ.

Further experience has shown that matters are not quite that simple. In breast cancer, removing the ovaries (oophorectomy) or irradiating the ovaries (a somewhat less effective method of achieving the same goal) induces remission in only about 30 percent of patients with breast cancer. This fact has given rise to a school of thought that some breast cancers (30 percent) are "hormone-dependent," whereas others (70 percent) are not, and this view gains strong support from tissue-culture studies showing that the cells of some breast cancers contain estrogen-receptors, whereas those of others do not. Another view holds that all breast cancers benefit to some extent from oophorectomy, and that the 30-percent distinction depends on our judgment as to whether the remission obtained has been really significant and sustained for a reasonable length of time. Various biochemical tests have been devised to predict in advance those patients who might benefit, and thus to avoid unnecessary surgery in those who might not, but so far with little real success. The clinician is still left in the empirical situation of "try and see." This is still good doctoring—the operation is a comparatively minor one, with a prospect that a fair proportion of patients might obtain real benefit.

The procedure is usually reserved for patients with disseminated disease, and the dramatic responders enjoy relief of bone pain and visible regression of metastases. This improvement may last six months or longer, but anything over a year is considered rather remarkable, and the disease inevitably recurs. Some surgeons advise oophorectomy at the time of mastectomy even when no known dissemination of disease is apparent, but the majority, basing their arguments on the fact that the benefit to be gained is always of limited duration, prefer to keep oophorectomy in reserve lest it be needed later.

When patients relapse after oophorectomy, they may respond again to removal of the adrenal glands (bilateral adrenalectomy), and, in the event of further relapse, to destruction of the pituitary gland (hypophysectomy), either by surgery or by implanting a radioactive source within the gland. Although benefit can still be obtained, these are all fairly major procedures, with their own risks and inherent morbidities, and they tend to be used not only to prolong life but also, and mainly, for the relief of distressing symptoms such as bone pain from skeletal metastases. The rationale behind these procedures is that some estrogen is produced in the adrenals, which will be removed by adrenalectomy, and some elsewhere, which will be dampened down by removing the pituitary. And, in passing, it is of interest to note that only those patients who have enjoyed a good response to oophorectomy are likely to benefit from adrenalectomy and hypophysectomy.

Suppression of estrogen can also be achieved by the giving of male hormone and other closely related anabolic steroids, such as testosterone propionate, and about the same proportion of breast-cancer patients, although not necessarily the same patients, show a good therapeutic response. More recently specific anti-estrogen drugs (Tamoxifen, Nafoxidine, Clomiphene) free of the virilizing side effects of the male hormones have become available and have been brought into clinical use, and again about the same proportion of breast cancer patients (although again not necessarily the same patients) derive some benefit.

So far so good. Any way of *suppressing* estrogen production is of real benefit to a minority, but a substantial minority, of patients with breast cancer. But *administration* of estrogens (the synthetic compound DES is usually used) also benefits about the same proportion of patients with breast cancer. To complicate matters even further, if a hormone is used with real benefit to the patient and the disease relapses, as it almost invariably will, a significant proportion of patients will then enjoy a period of further benefit by simply stopping the hormone, the so-called "withdrawal effect."

Because we do not know exactly how hormones act in breast cancer, this treatment is far from an exact science. However, clinical experience has established certain guidelines. In young pre-menopausal women with disseminated breast cancer oophorectomy is probably the treatment of first choice, with adrenalectomy and hypophysectomy held in reserve and used only for the relief of distressing symptoms. Such pre-menopausal patients might also be expected to benefit from estrogen suppression achieved by the administration of male hormones or anti-estrogen drugs, and a combination of oophorectomy and either an androgen or an anti-estrogen (or indeed both) would seem to offer the best prospects of success.

By contrast, in post-menopausal women (and again, of course, only those with disseminated breast cancer) DES appears to be the treatment of first choice.

In peri-menopausal women (within five years of the menopause) the ideal regime has still to be determined, and even between the clearly pre-menopausal and clearly post-menopausal groups there is a good deal of confusing overlap. Most surgeons of any experience can record instances of benefit following oophorectomy in post-menopausal women (although understandably, not in the aged), and also of post-menopausal women who respond to male hormones and pre-menopausal women who appear to respond to estrogens. So, although there are broad guidelines, we are reduced to a policy of altering the treatment according to response.

This fact in no way diminishes the value of the hormonal treatment of breast cancer. By varying a patient's endocrine status there is a reasonable chance of producing significant benefit for appreciable periods of time, and by switching the regimes, sometimes to "no regime," of extending that period of symptom-free time even further, and with none of the unpleasant side-effects associated with the alternative cytotoxic chemotherapy. Dr. George Beatson was knighted for building, organizing, and running a 2000-bed Red Cross hospital in Glasgow during the First World War. Posterity will surely accord him much greater recognition as the pioneer in the hormonal treatment of cancer.

We are on much firmer ground in the hormonal treatment of prostatic cancer, pioneered by Charles Huggins of Chicago, who was rightly awarded the Nobel Prize for his achievement. The viability and activity of the cells of the prostate gland depend upon the steady release of the male hormone testosterone from the cells of the testes. In eunuchs, the prostate, as a recognizable structure, all but disappears. Therefore if you remove the source of male hormone by castration (bilateral orchidectomy) or suppress it by overloading the system with female sex hormone (usually DES), a cancer of the prostate will regress. Furthermore, the response rate in this fairly common form of male cancer is much higher than the response rate in cancer of the breast, and the period of remission is usually far longer; so much so that, because this is predominantly a disease of the elderly, its hormonal control is usually sufficiently prolonged that having such an illness may make little or no difference to life expectancy.

With respect to the dosage of DES to be used, wide differences of opinion exist. If we listen to the biochemists, who can check the disappearance of testosterone from the circulating blood, only fractional doses, of the order of 0.1 to 1 milligram (mg) per day, are necessary. The recommendations of clinicians experienced in the treatment of human prostatic cancer patients are much larger: a common regime is 5 mg per day for the first month, 3 mg per day for the second month, and 1 mg per day indefinitely thereafter. This wide latitude in recommended dose can exist because DES, unlike any cytotoxic agent, is fundamentally a quite safe substance. In the higher dose ranges it can cause some nausea and breast discomfort, with nipple pigmentation and at times embarrassing breast enlargement, and certainly loss of libido and sexual potency, but most patients would agree that these are acceptable prices to pay to be free from a particularly painful form of cancer (it tends to metastasize to the bones). Prostatic cancer has a good biochemical marker to assess progress. It produces an enzyme, serum acid phosphatase—or, more specifically, tartrate-labile acid phosphatase—which can be easily measured in a blood sample. The concentration remains within a precise low range in health, and rises progressively in cancer of the prostate. A measured reduction in the levels is a clear, precise, and specific indication of therapeutic response.

The administration of DES has one potentially dangerous side-effect. It tends to lead to retention of sodium ions, and secondarily to water retention to keep the body's sodium-ion concentration within normal limits. This situation is analogous to pre-menstrual tension in the female. It is no problem for any reasonably healthy individual, but it can be a problem in those suffering from any moderate to severe degree of cardiac, respiratory, or renal impairment. In such situations overloading of the system with excess fluid can be dangerous. Preventing this requires restriction of dietary salt, the use of diuretics, and reduction of DES dosage, but these are all matters well within the province of any competent physician.

The majority of prostatic cancer patients respond to estrogens, but a few do not, and they tend to be in the younger age groups and to be individuals with more anaplastic, less well differentiated tumors, showing every other biochemical indication of malignancy except the "purposeful" rise in the serum acid phosphatase levels. Treatment in these circumstances is much more difficult. Adrenalectomy and hypophysectomy have been recommended, and have been shown to have some real but limited success. Local methods of treatment, such as external irradiation of the prostate or the implantation of radioactive seeds within the prostatic substance, enjoy some success. Palliative surgery in the form of transurethral prostatic resection, removing a fair mass of the tumor tissue, is very valuable in relieving obstructive urinary difficulties. Precisely because hormone-resistant tumor is almost by definition highly anaplastic, some response to cytotoxic chemotherapy can be obtained. But the sad truth is that if a patient with prostatic cancer fails to respond to estrogens (the exception, it must be stressed) his outlook is rather grim.

The lining of the uterus (the endometrium) is another target organ under hormonal control. During the first half of the menstrual cycle estrogen production invokes proliferative changes in the endometrium in a local, almost pseudo-neoplastic fashion; after ovulation in mid-cycle, the release of progesterone commands these young cells to mature and differentiate. It has been shown in experimental animals that the continuous administration of high doses of estrogens will relatively quickly produce frank uterine cancer. Thus many believe that cancer of the uterus (endometrial carcinoma) may be due to the unopposed action of a natural over-production of estrogens. In the late 1950s synthetic forms of progesterone, called progestogens, become available. There are now a whole variety of such compounds, of which Provera (medroxyprogesterone acetate) is a fairly typical and widely used example. With a background of knowledge about the hormonal control of the normal endometrial cycle, it could be predicted that administration of an overloading dose of progesterone might lead to maturation, differentiation, and some reversal to normal behavior of endometrial carcinoma cells. Clinical trials have established that this is indeed the case. Provera (and similar progestogens) will induce remission, sustained for an appreciable period of time, in around 35 or 40 percent of patients with endometrial cancer. This hormonal treatment need be used only in patients with disseminated disease, because in this variety of cancer the sign, abnormal vaginal bleeding, usually occurs very early, leading to swift diagnosis, and at that stage the results of purely local treatments, surgery and radiotherapy, can produce very high cure rates.

The kidney was not generally regarded as a hormonal target organ until the fortuitous discovery was made that the administration of estrogens to hamsters produces a significantly high incidence of kidney adenocarcinomas. In view of the success of hormonal treatment in other areas, this led to the proposal that progestogens, the natural counterbalance to estrogens, might have some value in human adenocarcinoma of the kidney. Clinical trials with Provera and related compounds were started, and, although it is now appreciated that the preliminary reports were over-optimistic, it is accepted that about 10 percent of patients with this form of cancer might expect some significant degree of benefit from this treatment sustained for a reasonable period of time.

One of the real successes of hormonal treatment occurs in a somewhat rare form of cancer, functioning adenocarcinomas (well-differentiated and usually papillary) of the thyroid gland. Like the cells of the normal thyroid, these malignant cells also produce the thyroid hormones, such as thyroxine. In other words, although malignant, they have retained a high degree of recognizable structure and function. The production of thyroxine is under the supervisory control of the pituitary, the gland at the base of the brain that masterminds the whole body-wide scenario. If the production of thyroxine falls, as measured by its concentration in the continuous monitoring of blood passing through the hypothalamus (another structure at the base of the brain), the pituitary immediately responds by releasing more thyroid stimulating hormone to boost production back to normal levels. On the other hand, if too much thyroxine is being produced (or at least detected) fewer such chemical telegraphic commands will be sent out. We can fool the pituitary computer by giving thyroxine to a patient with disseminated functioning thyroid cancer. The control commands then drop to near zero levels, and these thyroid-cancer slaves, no matter how far they have been disseminated, may cease to function, and may disappear.

Theoretical considerations about testicular cancer have evolved the thought that progestogens might inhibit these growths, and clinical trials are now in progress. Preliminary results suggest that some remission might be attained in about 30 percent of such patients, but it is too early to say whether the remission will be sustained for any appreciable period of time.

The ovary relays and supervises a whole complex of chemical compounds in the female that issue from the pituitary gland. Ovarian cancer, therefore, might be expected to be hormone-sensitive, but so far clinical trials have failed to demonstrate this in any convincing manner. It seems probable that we still have to decipher the correct hormonal combination to dampen down ovarian cell proliferation. It is also likely that the ovary consists of a whole spectrum of different target cells, and that what might restrain a cancer arising from one would have no effect on the cancers arising from the others.

The adrenal gland produces three main classes of hormones: the sex hormones (estrogens, androgens, and progesterone) in both men and women; the mineralocorticoids (concerned with salt conservation); and the glucocorticoids, concerned with carbohydrate metabolism, the control of the lymphatic system, and connective tissue in general. The release of the glucocorticoids is controlled by the release of adrenocorticotrophic hormone (ACTH) from the pituitary. Thus to obtain a glucocorticoid effect we may administer either a glucocorticoid or ACTH and let the adrenal do the job for us.

The glucocorticoids (cortisone, hydrocortisone, and their synthetic analogs prednisone, prednisole, dexamethazone, etc.) have an established place in cancer management. In general they produce an increased sense of well-being, and, although non-specific, such an effect may still be very valuable in general cancer treatment. Their more specific effect is on the lymphocytes. The administration of ACTH or any glucocorticoid (usually prednisone) will produce a sharp fall in the number of lymphocytes, and this is true whether the lymphocytes are normal or malignant. Therefore, the main value of glucocorticoids is in the management of lymphatic leukemias and the malignant lymphomas (Hodgkin's disease and the like). Prednisone, for instance, is often used as the drug of first choice for inducing remission in acute lymphatic leukemia, is frequently used for the same purpose in chronic lymphatic leukemia, and is an essential component of the combined regimes used in the management of the malignant lymphomas.

The glucocorticoids also exert a pronounced anti-inflammatory action. The total mass of any tumor consists of the volume of tumor cells plus the cells involved in the surrounding and intervening inflammatory reaction of the host. In certain situations the sheer size of any tumor can for mechanical reasons be highly dangerous, the typical example being compression of the brain by an intracranial tumor. In such situations the administration of a glucocorticoid (intravenous hydrocortisone for speed of action, or dexamethazone for power of action) can often be life-saving and tide the patient over until more effective measures can be initiated.

Therefore cortisone and related drugs are of specific value in the treatment of malignancies of the lymphatic system, and their antilymphocytic and anti-inflammatory actions can be of some help in the symptomatic management of many other forms of cancer. However, lymphocytic activity and the inflammatory reaction are important elements of the patient's own resistance, and attempts to constrain and restrain invasive tumor cells and to damp down these responses for short-term gain (except in the emergency situation already mentioned) is an exercise of dubious value.

In this chapter we have attempted to summarize the current status of the hormonal treatment of cancer. The situation is far from perfect. Many types of tumor are apparently totally unresponsive to hormonal manipulations, and even in cancers arising in organs under clear hormonal control only a proportion of the patients can expect to benefit. However, the total group contains two of the most common cancers of all, cancer of the breast and cancer of the prostate, so that the total benefit of hormonal treatment to mankind is enormous. Moreover, benefit is usually obtained without unpleasant side-effects. Thus, by the hormonal treatment of cancer we can achieve in many patients the goal of extending life in dignity and comfort. No doubt research will steadily extend the range and scope of this therapeutic approach in coming years.

9

The Treatment of Cancer by Immunotherapy

The human body has some very effective methods of protecting itself against cancer and other diseases. There is no doubt that these defenses overcome many incipient cancers and often prevent metastases from forming. Persons whose immune mechanisms are not operating effectively are especially susceptible to cancer as well as to other diseases. The idea that significant control of cancer can be achieved by making these natural protective mechanisms more effective, thus helping the body to help itself, is an appealing one, and for more than 80 years efforts to stimulate the immune system in order to achieve this result have been under way. Only recently, however, have these efforts been appreciated; because of a clearer understanding of their modes of action they now offer real promise of being used effectively.

This treatment of cancer is usually called *immunotherapy*, treatment by use of the immune mechanisms. The basic idea of immunotherapy is especially attractive because it involves fighting the disease by natural means, using the body's own defense mechanisms, and the danger of serious side effects of the treatment is accordingly small.

A successful outcome of any form of cancer treatment depends on our ability to distinguish the tumor from normal tissues, and then to destroy it. At its simplest level, the surgical excision of a localized tumor with minimal damage to surrounding tissues exploits this difference. Radiation treatment in which the electromagnetic energy is focussed to maximum intensity on the tumor area is essentially another local form of treatment. Chemotherapy is more selectively destructive to rapidly growing tumors than to slowly growing ones, and, as we have seen, it enjoys its only real predictable successes in such situations. What we desperately need is some agent that will select with great precision only tumor cells, no matter where they are situated, and then selectively destroy them.

It is difficult to design such an agent, but in fact the whole complicated machinery, from the mechanisms necessary for the immediate identification of a "foreign invader" as "not-self" to the rapid manufacture of a battery of weapons quite specific to their target, already exists in the immune system.

This exquisite system responds immediately to an antigen (any foreign material producing the signal "not-self") by the rapid mobilization of specific defenses. These are of two types: antibodies, which are proteins called immunoglobulins that are specifically designed to lock precisely onto the antigen and to trigger off its destruction by the ultimate chemical weapon, the complex of proteins called *complement*, and special cells, lymphocytes that are no different in appearance from other lymphocytes, but are produced by the millions as a special clone to seek out and destroy this specific antigen. Thus we have already in existence a highly sophisticated system with the capability we seek.

The trouble is that a tumor is not a foreign invader, but is a true native-born cell of the patient that has undergone a few changes such as to cause it to behave in an abnormal way. Almost all of the molecules that make up the cells of the tumor are identical with those in the cells of the normal tissues of the patient, and those molecules cannot act as antigens in that person. Fortunately, however, the few changes that are characteristic of the tumor involve molecules that are different from those that are normally present at birth, and hence can function as antigens in the patient. The tumor cells accordingly evoke a weak antigenic response, and the patient begins to manufacture antibody molecules that can combine with the antigens of the tumor cells and thus identify these cells as not-self, and set into action the whole complex immune process. Detection of the antigen-antibody response in the circulating blood can be used to diagnose the presence of some kinds of cancer. Moreover, the immune response is often so vigorous as to overcome the incipient cancer.

Some patients, such as those who receive kidney transplants from a non-identical-twin donor, are given drugs that suppress the immune system. These patients show a high incidence of spontaneous cancers as the years go by, and this high incidence can be explained as resulting from the suppression of the mechanism of immune surveillance. Moreover, there are published reports of rather rare but intriguing examples of the spontaneous remission of cancers, sometimes even far advanced cancers, following some powerful stimulation of the immune system.

The general view is that the immune system acts as a police force, continually patrolling the tissues, detecting any miscreants and then destroying them, and in this way keeping the body free from cancer. Every now and then this protective system breaks down and a cancer becomes established, but even then it is believed that the immune system plays an important part in retarding progressive growth and in picking off wandering tumor cells that could be on the way to cause trouble elsewhere. Thus, enhancing the immune system could play an important part in general cancer treatment, and any measure that depresses the immune system (and unfortunately cancer chemotherapy does just that) decreases the effectiveness of treatment.

The beginnings of cancer immunotherapy date back to some remarkable observations by physicians and surgeons in the United States and Europe that were published between 1866 and 1900. It was observed that a number of patients with far advanced cancer who developed acute bacterial infections with fever and inflammation—especially streptococcal infections (erysipelas) and staphylococcal or other pyogenic (pus-forming) infections—recovered from their cancers. The streptococcal infections led to the most dramatic disappearance of even very large inoperable cancers, whereas the staphylococcal or pyogenic infections produced the largest number of permanent regressions. This difference may have been the result of the facts that the erysipelas infections were of short duration and the others lasted longer and could stimulate the immune defenses for a long enough time to permit them to destroy all of the tumor cells.

These observations led Dr. William B. Coley, then (in 1896) a young surgeon in New York City, to inoculate advanced cancer patients with cultures of streptococcus from erysipelas patients. His first case failed to develop erysipelas until the fourth culture was tried; the tumor then disappeared. After a year of such trials, without great success, Coley began using heat-killed or filtered vaccines produced from streptococci and another non-pathogenic bacterium (now called *Serratia marcescens*). This mixed vaccine became known as Coley's Mixed Toxins or Coley's Fluid. Injections of the preparation produced reactions (fever, chills), but so little was known about the best ways to prepare and to administer these vaccines that the results were quite variable and the treatment never achieved widespread use. Also, just after Coley began this work x-rays and radium were discovered, and interest in their use in treating cancer soon became so great as to cause other new treatments to be ignored.

Nevertheless, recent studies of the results of Coley's treatment (International Cancer Conference, London, 1978) have shown that of 894 patients with various types of cancer who received the Coley treatment 426 recovered and were traced 5 to 80 years later; 237 of the 426 were inoperable advanced cases when Coley began treating them. Although a bibliography on Coley's method lists 368 papers in the period 1893 to 1977, most present-day oncologists (cancer specialists) ignore this therapy.

Scientists are now beginning to understand the mechanisms of action of Coley's vaccines, concurrent infections, and other immunostimulants, such as vitamin C (Chapter 15). They exert a powerful stimulating action on the immune system, causing increased production of immunoglobulins and lymphocytes, and this triggered awareness and increased efficiency are sufficient to swamp some of the highly susceptible tumors, leaving others apparently uninfluenced. It is interesting that among the patients who showed a dramatic response to this kind of therapy there was a high proportion with very rapidly proliferating tumors. Again, as with radiotherapy and chemotherapy, the more vicious the tumor, the greater is the chance of being able to do something useful about it.

A few investigators are now using mixed bacterial vaccines prepared from bacteria that cause serious or fatal infections in immunosuppressed cancer patients in order to increase their resistance to these infections and also to the cancer. The preliminary results are encouraging. Injections of these vaccines prior to radiotherapy or chemotherapy as well as after these immunosuppressive treatments may well have value.

Several other methods of stimulating the immune system into high activity are also under trial. These consist of repeated inoculation with BCG (attenuated tuberculosis vaccine) or injections of other non-specific antigens. The side effects of BCG therapy are, however, often disagreeable. A few dramatic responses have been reported, but we are a long way from talking about cancer cures by such means. Probably their use will become established as a supportive measure alongside more definitive treatment, for instance, adjuvant immunotherapy soon after curative surgery in the hope of mopping up any residual wayward cells with more efficiency than usual.

Another way of increasing immunocompetence is to make sure that the lymphocytes are saturated with ascorbic acid, and therefore are able to perform their scavenging tasks more efficiently. There are also some reports in the scientific literature that an increased intake of vitamin A increases lymphocytic immunocompetence. Thus a regime consisting of the lymphocytes being brought to peak efficiency by adequate intakes of vitamin A and vitamin C and periodically boosted to even greater efficiency by the use of some non-specific stimulant such as a bacterial vaccine may be found to be the best method of employing the immune system in cancer treatment.

The more direct methods of employing the immune system, by inoculating the patient with sterilized tumor cells or tumor cell antigen extracts or with anti-tumor antibodies obtained by inoculating tumor cell suspensions into some intermediate animal species, have not so far enjoyed any great success, but research is being actively pursued in all these fields and advances can be anticipated. At the present time it seems to us that the best way of using immunotherapy and stimulating the body's natural defenses against cancer is by the intake of proper amounts of vitamin C and by other nutritional measures, as discussed in later chapters of this book.

10

Some Unconventional Forms of Cancer Treatment

By the label "unconventional" we designate forms of cancer treatment that have not gained general acceptance in medical practice. These unconventional forms of cancer treatment are not universally and dramatically effective, and usually their alleged modes of action have never been scientifically explained. It is fundamental to medical reasoning that if we do not understand how an agent influences a disease, then any reports of changes induced in the disease by the agent tend to be dismissed as anecdotal rubbish.

In digressing to mention unconventional forms of cancer treatment we are conscious of our entry into a murky area, thickly populated by cranks, frauds, charlatans, and misguided persons but also including some honest, far-sighted, and original investigators who were striving to contribute to the effort of controlling a disease that is responsible for a major part of the misery of the world's people. The failure of conventional treatment of cancer in many millions of patients has created an eager willingness to believe almost any therapeutic claim, and over the years many hundreds of such claims have been made. Because of the relatively slow development of many human cancers, many such claims can acquire spurious substance.

We are well aware that the "placebo effect" and even worse the "observer anticipation effect" can exist in cancer, as in every other malady. If any treatment, even a carefully measured dose of distilled water, is given with conviction to cancer patients, a fraction of the patients will swear that they have benefitted, and their therapists, if they sincerely believe in the regime, will be equally convinced that some degree of benefit has accrued. These are very human reactions, not to be stigmatized as charlatanry.

However, in cancer the scope for placebo and anticipation effects is somewhat limited; with rare exceptions, we are dealing with a relentlessly progressive disease, with a drastically clearly defined end point, death, which restricts such subjective imaginative distortion.

Therefore if we reject the obviously fraudulent claims of outrageous quacks, we are still left with a number of unconventional cancer treatments to consider, and it might be prudent to keep an open mind. Some of these unconventional forms of cancer treatment have been advocated by persons who may have discovered some means of altering the whole tumor-host relationship in a favorable direction.

Mention has already been made of the pioneer work of Coley and his Coley's Fluid, which for a period enjoyed world-wide popularity as an anticancer remedy and then fell into disrepute. Only now are we beginning to understand its mode of action; it is a powerful stimulant of the immune system, capable of wiping out some susceptible cancers. And if it can wipe out a few, logic suggests that it should be retarding the remainder in varying degrees. Coley was elected an Honorary Fellow of the Royal College of Surgeons of London in 1935, six months before his death; yet within two decades the American Cancer Society had included Coley's Mixed Toxins in their quackery list, *New and Unproven Methods of Cancer Treatment*.

Then there is the intriguing Krebiozen story. Dr. Andrew Ivy, nominated by the American Medical Association to be their representative at the Nuremberg atrocity trials on the basis of his high professional reputation, put this reputation at stake by his advocacy of Krebiozen as a form of cancer treatment. Krebiozen was a white powder "chemically separated from horses' serum after stimulation of their cell network by the injection of *Actinomyces bovis*." It was claimed to be a lipopolysaccharide, which might have acted, when injected into patients, as an immunostimulant, but the Food and Drug Administration reported that it had been identified as creatine (the compound N-methyl-N-guanylglycine, a normal constituent of muscle), which could not be expected to be effective against cancer. Ivy and his associates were tried for fraud in selling the drug as an agent for suppressing cancer. Although they were found to be not guilty, Ivy's reputation was ruined. Reputable physicians testified to the apparent efficacy of the substance in some patients, and we have the opinion that there is the possibility that in these patients it was acting as an immunostimulant.

There is also the interesting story of Dr. Max Gerson, the German immigrant to New York State who set up a successful clinic devoted to the dietary treatment of cancer. The diet was basically raw fruits and vegetables, with special emphasis on drinking each day many glasses of freshly expressed juices of oranges, grapefruit, apples, grapes, tomatoes, carrots, and green leaves. This diet contains very large amounts of vitamin C, vitamin A, various B vitamins, minerals, and other nutrients. There is little doubt that this diet and other features of Gerson's treatment, such as the detoxification of the body by frequent enemas, appear to have been of benefit to some cancer patients, as described in his 1958 book *A Cancer Therapy: Results of Fifty Cases*. It is regrettable that in 1946 a bill including a provision for research on the Gerson treatment was narrowly defeated in the United States Senate. Since then the National Cancer Institute and the American Cancer Society have ignored nutrition as a factor in the prevention and treatment of cancer almost completely; only recently has the U.S. Congress allocated money to support research in this field, and the agencies that make the grants to interested investigators continue to be reluctant to support any but the most pedestrian research projects in this backward field of science and medicine.

Dr. Gerson died in 1959. During recent years his cancer treatment or a treatment incorporating its major features has been used in several clinics. No significant accounts of the results obtained in the treatment of patients have been published, however, and there is still much uncertainty about how great the value of this kind of nutritional therapy may be. It is our opinion that proper nutritional therapy will ultimately be accepted as having great value as an adjunct to the conventional treatments.

The use of Laetrile or amygdalin for the treatment of cancer is under investigation and vigorous discussion at the present time. Laetrile is L-mandelonitrile-β-glucuronic acid, $C_{14}H_{15}NO_7$, a compound patented in 1958 by Krebs and Krebs of the John Beard Memorial Foundation of San Francisco. It can be made synthetically from mandelonitrile and glucose and can also be obtained from amygdalin by hydrolysis and oxidation. Amygdalin is a more complex substance, D-mandelonitrile-β-D-glucosido-6-β-D-glucoside, $C_{20}H_{27}NO_{11}$, which occurs in seeds of *Rosaceae*, especially almonds and apricot seeds, from which it can be obtained by extraction with alcohol. It is our understanding that the substance now referred to as Laetrile and used in the treatment of cancer is amygdalin. These two substances contain a nitrile (cyanide) group, and hydrogen cyanide is released by them under certain conditions. It has been suggested that cyanide is released more effectively in cancer cells than in normal cells, and that the cancer cells are thus preferentially killed, but the evidence for such an action is not strong. Laetrile treatment has been claimed to improve the general health of cancer patients and to increase their survival times. It is estimated that as many as 300,000 people have received this treatment. Laetrile treatment has been strongly opposed by the American Medical Association, the National Cancer Institute, the Food and Drug Administration, and the American Cancer Society.

We have examined a large number of documents about Laetrile. We have not seen any evidence that would permit us to make the definite statement that Laetrile has significant value for cancer patients. On the other hand, we have not seen any evidence that would permit us to make the definite statement that Laetrile has no value at all. There is the possibility that it has a little value. It is not a very dangerous drug—it is far less poisonous than aspirin, for example. But it is rather expensive, and it is our opinion at the present time that it is not worth while to spend the money and go to the effort necessary to obtain Laetrile.

The problem is complicated by the fact that Laetrile treatment of cancer patients as practiced by various physicians involves much more than the injection or oral ingestion of Laetrile. These physicians often prescribe vitamin C, usually in the amount 10 grams per day. We are convinced that this intake of vitamin C has value—in fact, great value—for essentially every cancer patient. Moreover, the patient is put on a vegetarian diet, a regime resembling that of Max Gerson, and he is given digestive enzymes and large amounts of vitamin A, other vitamins, and minerals. This part of the treatment also probably has real value in improving the health of the patient and controlling his disease. We think that what is called the Laetrile treatment of cancer is of benefit to most of the patients, but we rather doubt that the Laetrile itself contributes significantly to its effectiveness.

The truth about cancer at the present time is that we do not have one single agent or treatment that can be relied upon to cure every patient with cancer or even every patient with one kind of cancer. The conventional methods of cancer treatment usually fail; should we not now carefully investigate those unconventional methods that claim a few successes?

First, of course, the truly fraudulent claims must be discarded. But novel methods of therapy should not be rejected just because they are novel, or because they run counter to some generally accepted belief (which may be just bias), or because we do not understand the mechanism of the proposed treatment, or because it has come from an unconventional source. It is essential, if progress is to be made in the attack on cancer, that the people involved, and especially those in the National Cancer Institute and the American Cancer Society, strive to open their minds to new ideas.

Then, having identified those measures, both conventional and unconventional, that can offer some modicum of help to cancer patients, it should be possible to link all these measures together into combined regimes that will provide genuine help to everyone who has the misfortune of developing this disease.

PART III

A RATIONAL APPROACH TO THE TREATMENT OF CANCER

11

Controlling Cancer

As mentioned in an earlier chapter, the two fundamental characteristics of the malignant cell are autonomous proliferation and invasiveness. All conventional forms of cancer treatment have concentrated on the cell-proliferative aspect, and the basic principle of treatment has been that if all these abnormally proliferating cells could be destroyed the patient would be freed from cancer. Thus these renegade cells are "cut out, burned out, poisoned, or otherwise destroyed" in the hope of effecting a cure, and this effort has been successful in only about one-third of all cancer patients. It has failed in the other two-thirds, and although various stratagems may succeed in delaying the progress of the disease for a while, eventually these patients die from their disease.

To cure only one third is a pretty miserable achievement, and, although marginal progress continues to be made, the way ahead has seemed to be frustratingly blocked by an impenetrable iron curtain. Two-thirds of the patients are not helped because the proliferating cells have already spread beyond the reach of the surgeon's knife or the range of the radiotherapist's beams, or are not proliferating fast enough to be poisoned out of existence by any drugs that have been devised without poisoning the patient out of existence at the same time.

For some years we have stood virtually alone in recommending an alternative strategy, which to us seems to hold out far more promise of success (Cameron, 1966; Cameron and Pauling, 1973). The alternative strategy is to concentrate on the other main characteristic of malignancy: invasiveness. Invasiveness, the ability of tumor cells to erode their way through tissues, ulcerate through surfaces, and enter the lymphatic and blood circulatory systems to set up metastases elsewhere, is responsible for all the dangerous features of malignancy. Stopping invasiveness would eliminate these dangers. Invasiveness is a property possessed only by cancer cells, and therefore provides a specific target for therapeutic attack.

Let us consider what would happen if we could suddenly disarm malignant cells and render them non-invasive. In the first place, this treatment would be available for all patients with cancer, irrespective of the extent of their disease. It would convert the existing destructive and invasive metastases into benign relatively innocuous non-invasive tumors. This would create a truce-like situation, with the patient having to live with his cancers, but, unlike the earlier situation, with the cancers having to behave and conform within the patient. In practice the benefits to the patient could be even greater.

In order to suggest ways of controlling malignant invasiveness we have need to understand the mechanism of its action. Tumor cells steadily release enzymes that are able to erode a way through almost every barrier placed in their path. The primary barrier is the ground substance, the ubiquitous intercellular cement mentioned in our preface and in Chapter 1, and indeed secondary barriers, whether they consist of sheets of cells such as in mucous membranes or the walls of blood vessels, consist of nothing more than specialized cells stuck together by this ground substance. The chemistry of the ground substance is a fairly complex subject that does not need to be discussed here. We can simply say that it owes its high viscosity and structural cohesion to the presence of certain very large long-chain polymers, macromolecules built up of endlessly repeating relatively simple molecules. Tumor cells release an enzyme, hyaluronidase, that has the specific ability to break up these large polymers into shorter and shorter units. The effect of this is to liquefy the ground substance in the immediate vicinity of the tumor cells, giving them room to move and to push forward, always preceded by an area of change in their micro-environment. The malignant cells are no longer stuck in highly viscous cement, as are their non-malignant brethren. They have created their own less restricting micro-environment, and they can create this new environment wherever they go. Ahead of them the ground substance disappears, and the organized normal structures simply fall apart as the cementing substance is attacked by the enzymes.

By controlling this invasiveness of the malignant tumors their spread would be brought under control. But the benefits could be much greater. All cells, normal or malignant, gain their essential nourishment by a process of diffusion, the seeping of these essential nutrients through the walls of the capillaries and through the intervening ground substance. If these intervening barriers are first eroded away by the invasive enzymes the process of diffusion is very much enhanced, and this is the reason why tumor cells always acquire the lion's share of the available food. This is the explanation of the well-known clinical situation of a tumor thriving in a patient who becomes progressively more and more emaciated. Hence if we were able to stop invasiveness we would also stop the selective routing of food to the tumor, and this would markedly retard its growth. Furthermore, because many very rapidly growing tumors are existing at the very far limits of diffusion with only a few primitive blood vessels having had time to form, a sudden cut off in this diffusion mechanism could have drastic effects on the tumor, causing millions of over-stretched cells to die abruptly from suffocation and starvation. It is necessary to be careful in the latter circumstance, as the sheer size of the tumor may pose a problem. Killing a small tumor or scattered small deposits of tumor would be tantamount to cure, but killing a large volume of tumor at one time would present the body's metabolic system with the tremendous overload of dispos-ing of the waste products of several hundred grams of dead tumor tissue. Thus a "cure" situation might result in the death of the patient with extensive tumors. However, we believe that the chance that this would occur is small, being significant only for those rare patients with extremely rapidly growing tumors that are extending themselves to the very outer limits of nutritional survival.

In general, the effect of interfering with this mechanism would be to stop all further invasiveness, and to slow down markedly the rate of tumor growth. This would be a significant advance in the treatment of cancer.

In addition, there is the possibility that controlling invasiveness would also control to some extent the unrestrained cell division characteristic of malig-nancy. We have postulated (Cameron, 1966; Cameron and Pauling, 1973) that in normal tissues the tendency to proliferate is held in check because the cells are embedded in viscous ground substance. In order to proliferate the cells release enzymes to attack the ground substance and remove this restraint, thus gaining space for an increased number of cells. Proliferation may stop when the release of hyaluronidase stops and the environment returns to its normal restraining pattern. If this idea about hyaluronidase and cell proliferation is correct, control of the release of hyaluronidase by malignant cells would not only decrease the invasiveness of the cancer but would also decrease its tendency toward cell division, slowing down the growth of the tumor and perhaps even stopping it. Accordingly, control of the liberation of hyaluroni-dase would be a significant step forward in the treatment of cancer (Cameron, 1966).

How might this be done? One approach is to make the ground substance more resistant to the enzymes released by the tumor. This can be achieved locally by treatment with high-energy radiation, and systematically by the administration of various hormones. It is a striking fact that the hormones that have been found to be of some use in the management of human cancers (estrogens, androgens, thyroxine, and cortisone, but not progesterone) have been found also to possess this property of increasing the resistance of the ground substance to attack (references are given in Cameron, 1966).

Some drugs are known that block the action of tumor hyaluronidase; they have not, however, been used as anti-cancer agents (for references see Cameron, 1966).

Our own interest has focused in part upon a natural feedback mechanism and the question as to how it might best be employed in the control of cancer. This feedback mechanism depends upon the existence of a natural inhibitor of hyaluronidase (physiological hyaluronidase inhibitor, PHI). In health, the concentration of PHI in the blood serum remains within a fairly narrow range. In cancer (and in some other diseases, an important point with potential therapeutic implications) the serum PHI concentration invariably rises, but to a variable extent. One of our basic approaches has been that if serum PHI could be boosted to the maximum possible level in every cancer patient very significant improvements in cancer treatment might result. Moreover, many or all malignant tumors liberate the enzyme collagenase, which attacks the collagen fibrils in the ground substance and thus weakens it. Those measures that can prevent attack on the ground substance or can strengthen it should help in controlling the disease. As is discussed in the following chapters, we believe that improved nutrition, and especially the use of vitamin C in proper amounts, can be effective in these ways.

12

Spontaneous Regression in Cancer

Sometimes a patient suffering from cancer begins, for no obvious reason, to improve. If the manifestations of his disease become less serious for a time he is said to have experienced a spontaneous remission, and if these manifestations disappear he is said to have experienced a spontaneous regression or even a spontaneous cure of the disease. It is likely, of course, that these remissions or regressions are not truly spontaneous, but instead have a cause, which might be the stimulation of the patient's immune system when he contracts an infection, such as erysipelas (Chapter 9), or changes his diet. The number of true spontaneous regressions of cancer that have been reported is usually given as 200 or 300 (Everson and Cole, 1966), but the number must in fact be much larger, because such a regression that occurred while the patient was undergoing treatment would be attributed to the treatment. Spontaneous regressions have been observed not only for patients with early malignant lesions but also for those with the most advanced disease.

Evidence about the occurrence of spontaneous regressions combines with other evidence to strengthen the belief that the natural protective mechanisms of the human body operate to overcome many malignant tumors. For example, cervical cytology (the Pap test) indicates that about 15 percent of women have "positive smears" at some time in their lives—that is, cells that show signs of malignancy—but only about 0.37 percent die of cancer of the cervix. This means that cancer of the cervix is a far commoner disease than we usually think it to be, but in 39 cases out of 40 the disease is controlled. Also, in many European hospitals meticulous autopsies are performed without regard to the cause of death, and these autopsies reveal a remarkably high incidence of cancers that were never suspected in life. For some cancers the number of these unrevealed cases is far greater than the number of revealed cases. For example, cancer of the thyroid and cancer of the pancreas are found to be 30 or 40 times as common in autopsy findings as are presented in the doctor's office. Autopsy cancer of the prostate increases steadily with increasing age until after age 75 it is found in every second male, yet only about 2 percent of males die of prostate cancer.

What are these mysterious cancers that turn up in such profusion in the dead but seem to have refrained from causing trouble during life? The tumors are usually small, but when they are looked at through the microscope they are seen to have essentially all the characteristics of a growing invasive cancer. Cancer is therefore far more common than we usually realize, and not such a vicious disease as is commonly thought, except when it gets out of control. The great majority of cancers are held in check by the body; they grow for a while, then regress and disappear, and it is only an occasional one that escapes from control and forms a progressive cancer.

It seems likely that, even in well-established cancers, "spontaneous regression" could be playing a more important part in treatment than we have realized in the past. If a cancer patient is treated and then lives for five years in good health, it is natural to assume that the treatment is responsible for this happy outcome. But this is not necessarily so. Almost every surgeon can remember carrying out resections that, for technical reasons, were less than adequate, and yet being gratified to find that the inadequately treated patient is still alive and in apparent good health many years later. There is increasing awareness that the doctor is not the only factor involved in the treatment situation, and that we have to rely a good deal upon nature to back up our efforts. Thus it is often good surgery to remove the main tumor even when it is known or strongly suspected that spread beyond the field of possible removal has already taken place. We then rely upon the immune system or natural resistance to destroy the remaining malignant cells. This sort of action can be seen quite strikingly in some patients with kidney cancer that has already spread to the lungs. The diseased kidney is removed, and sometimes the lung metastases then wither away and disappear completely. This, it must be stressed, is a very rare occurrence, but the fact that it can occur at all is truly remarkable.

When one talks of spontaneous regressions one usually thinks of the patient with hopelessly advanced disease, who, without any treatment, suddenly starts to get better, and may continue to get better until he is completely well. These near-miracles are extremely rare, but some hundreds of such instances have now been thoroughly documented. Spontaneous regression teaches us that doctors and their treatments are not all-powerful, and that there exists in every one of us a mechanism with the potential to cure cancer, working alongside whatever treatment is adopted. It is regrettable that it is not completely effective in every patient. A goal for cancer research is to find the ways to make this mechanism more effective.

13

Host Resistance
to Cancer

One need not be a cancer specialist to appreciate that not all cancers grow at the same speed. This may be because some tumors are more aggressive than others or because some patients are more resistant to cancer than others. Probably a combination of these two factors is at work in every patient.

We may not be able to do much about the inherent aggressiveness of different tumors, but it would be helpful if we could make every patient as resistant as possible to his disease. We consider in this chapter the factors that are associated with increased resistance to cancer. Many of these factors are unknown, but enough are known to give a few broad guidelines.

First we may consider age. The cancers of childhood and adolescence tend to grow rather quickly, whereas the cancers of the very elderly tend to grow quite slowly, with in between a gradual decrease of the rate of growth of the common cancers of adulthood and middle-age. These are only general trends, with exceptions occurring at every age.

Then there is the general constitution, a concept difficult to define. A patient with cancer and cardiac failure is liable to die sooner than a patient with cancer and a healthy heart, and the presence of any debilitating illness may make a person somewhat more liable to develop cancer and after it has developed to be less resistant to it. Patients do differ from one another quite markedly. It is possible to have two apparently identical patients receiving identical treatment, and to have one die in a matter of months from disseminated disease and the other live so long as to qualify as having been cured. There must be some constitutional explanation for this.

It is possible to inbreed experimental animals to produce strains that have a very high incidence of "spontaneous" cancers, that is, cancers that arise without any obvious external cause. It is also possible that some similar genetic factors are at work in the human population, although with cancer such a common disease it is nearly impossible to trace any hereditary factor, except in a few striking instances. Thus women with a strong family history of breast cancer among close blood relatives (mother, grandmother, sisters) are more likely to develop breast cancer than are other women and, moreover, are likely to develop it at a younger age. However, we are still a long way from genetic counselling to prevent cancer.

Among the factors associated with resistance to cancer the most striking one is *encapsulation,* the walling off of the tumor in a dense meshwork of fibrous tissue. This covers the whole spectrum from individuals with very rapidly growing highly invasive tumors where attempts at encapsulation are virtually non-existent, to the other end of the scale, the atrophic scirrhous tumors, which are very slow-growing tumors practically trapped in almost impenetrably dense scar tissue. It is not known whether the very anaplastic tumors are so aggressive that they completely obliterate this defensive reaction, or whether all tumors have the same inherent aggressiveness, but some are restrained by the power of this defensive response. The second interpretation is the more hopeful one.

Either way, this is a constitutional response, with a constant effect throughout the body. The amount of fibrosis (new scar tissue) is the same around the primary tumor and every one of its metastases, no matter where they are located, but, of course, the really atrophic scirrhous tumors may produce no metastases at all, because this defense reaction is so powerful and so successful.

Then there are the lymphocytes, the wandering policemen of the immune system, and a few other cells, such as macrophages, that perform a scavenging role. It has long been known that the degree of lymphocytic infiltration, the number of aggressive lymphocytes congregating in and around a tumor (as can readily be seen on a microscope slide) bears a close relation to the outlook. In patients with the most aggressive tumors lymphocytes are scanty or absent, whereas in the very slow-growing tumors lymphocytes are so abundant that they may dominate the whole microscopic appearance. This, too, is a constitutional response, with a rather similar degree of lymphocytic infiltration around the primary tumor and all its metastases. Most experts in this field agree that a good lymphocytic response indicates high patient resistance, and no one can doubt that a good lymphocytic response is associated with slow growth of the tumor and a much better outlook for the patient.

A good lymphocytic response is not confined to the actual tumor; it can be seen also in the regional lymph nodes draining the affected area, and it is assumed with a reasonable degree of confidence that these reactive lymph nodes are filtering off and destroying any wandering tumor cells that happen to come their way. As was mentioned in Chapter 7, it is a pity that cancer chemotherapy, whatever its undoubted advantages in certain situations, is particularly destructive to all lymphocytes.

These are the powerful local defensive reactions of the body against malignant invasive growth. There are also other factors of a more general nature, involving the immune system. Although immunotherapy for human cancer has not yet lived up to expectations, there is no doubt that the immune system is at work in every cancer patient, restraining his tumor to a greater or smaller degree. Here we have to consider the immunoglobulins, large protein molecules of considerable complexity, and manufactured to a special blueprint that will enable them to identify the malignant cells and to set in motion the sequence of events that culminates in their destruction.

There are various well-established techniques to measure the immunocompetence of individuals—that is, their ability to produce new lymphocytes on demand, the scavenging power of their macrophages, their production of specific immunoglobulins, and the strength of the different components of the complement system.

When these tests are carried out on patients with cancer the almost invariable finding is that their immunocompetence is markedly and sometimes severely depressed. Restoring their immunocompetence to normal levels should help to control their disease.

Another constitutional factor is the whole hormonal background of the individual. In Chapter 8 we discussed the hormonal treatment of certain cancers. We accept for the most part the widely held view that this treatment has its major value for those cancers involving the hormonal target tissue. The analysis of various hormonal breakdown products in the urine has shown that some individuals have what is described as a favorable steroid environment, whereas others have an unfavorable steroid environment, and that the general resistance to cancer is significantly higher in the former than in the latter. To repeat what was briefly mentioned in Chapter 8, the hormones that have been found useful in certain cancers, the estrogens, the androgens, cortisone, and thyroxine, all change the ground substance from an amorphous to a more fibrillar pattern, making it more resistant to the erosive effects of tumor hyaluronidase and therefore to tumor invasiveness.

Finally, as mentioned earlier, there is the possibility that the level of hyaluronidase inhibitor in the blood and tissues might play an important part in determining the progress of any cancer. Thus, although the picture is incomplete, we know many factors that may increase a patient's resistance to cancer. How some of these factors might be harnessed and brought into the realm of practical therapeutics is the subject of later chapters.

14

Vitamin C

Vitamin C is closely related to both scurvy and cancer. Scurvy is the disease that results from a deficiency in the intake of vitamin C. A person who receives none of this vitamin becomes seriously ill and soon dies. The relationship to cancer is much more complex, and much more important in the modern world, in which scurvy is rare and cancer is a scourge.

Vitamin C may turn out to be the most important of all nutrients in the control of cancer, but others are also important. Good nutrition, which means the exclusion from the diet of harmful substances as well as the inclusion of beneficial ones, can decrease the incidence of cancer significantly. Although much has been learned about nutrition and also about cancer during the last 100 years, there is still much more to be learned. It is encouraging that recently the U.S. Congress has taken action to increase the amount of research in this field.

A brief discussion of foods and nutrition is given in Appendix II. Many of the constituents of foods are essential to good health. Among these nutrients the vitamins may be considered to be especially important.

After many of his men had died of scurvy in 1536, the French explorer Jacques Cartier, at a site near the present city of Quebec, learned from the Indians that this disease could be prevented and treated by drinking a tea made from the leaves and bark of the arborvitae tree. The value of citrus fruits for preventing scurvy was also recognized early, especially by the Scottish physician James Lind, who in 1747 carried out an experiment with twelve patients severely ill with scurvy. He placed them all on the same diet, except for one or another of certain reputed remedies. Two patients received two oranges and one lemon a day, and the others received cider or vinegar or certain other substances. At the end of six days the two who had received the citrus fruits were well, whereas the others remained ill.

The ravages of scurvy among the early sea voyagers were terrible. For example, during his voyage of discovery of the sea route from Lisbon around Africa to India, 9 July 1497 to 20 May 1498, the Portuguese navigator Vasco da Gama lost 100 of his crew of 160 to scurvy. The supply of fresh fruit and vegetables ran out, and the sailors lived almost entirely on biscuits, salt beef, and salt pork, which provide essentially no vitamin C. During the next few months they were protected by using up the supply of ascorbate stored in their tissues, especially the adrenals and spleen. When this supply was exhausted, first in those who had been poorly nourished at the start of the voyage and later in the better-nourished ones, scurvy set in. The scorbutic sailor showed lassitude and then extreme prostration, swollen, tender, and bleeding gums, foul breath, a tendency to bruise easily, internal bleeding caused by broken blood vessels in the muscles and other tissues, weakness of the joints, profound exhaustion, diarrhea, and pulmonary and kidney troubles leading to coma, collapse, and death.

Pure L-ascorbic acid, vitamin C, was first prepared in 1928 by Albert Szent-Györgyi, but it was not until 1932 that his substance was shown to be vitamin C. Within a short time the value of large intakes of ascorbic acid in improving health began to be recognized. The pure substance became available in drug stores, and dietary supplements of vitamin C and other vitamins were soon being used by many people.

It is believed that about 5 milligrams of vitamin C per day is enough to prevent scurvy in most people, but larger amounts are required for really good health. The intake recommended for adults by the Food and Nutrition Board is 45 mg per day.

The various manifestations of scurvy, mentioned above, emphasize the importance of vitamin C to the proper functioning of the human body. The fact that as little as 5 mg (one five-thousandth of an ounce) per day is enough to prevent scurvy in most people shows how powerful this substance is. Yet, even though such minute doses have a profound physiological effect, vitamin C is not a dangerous substance. In the medical literature it is described as virtually non-toxic. Human beings have been given as much as 150 grams (g), one-third of a pound, of sodium ascorbate by injection or intravenous infusion without any serious side-effects. People have also taken even larger amounts by mouth without serious side-effects, and others have ingested 20 g per day for years without apparent damage, but rather with benefit to their health. Among these persons are patients treated by Dr. Fred R. Klenner of Reidsville, North Carolina, who has published a number of papers on the value of a high intake of vitamin C for the achievement of good health and for the treatment of various diseases. The only side-effect that occurs with much frequency is diarrhea, which is discussed in a later chapter of this book. Ascorbic acid is no more toxic than ordinary sugar (sucrose) and is less toxic than common salt, and far less toxic than aspirin or other drugs. There is no reported case of the death or severe illness of any person from ingesting too large an amount of ascorbic acid.

Vitamin C is found in many foods. Some foods, such as green peppers, red peppers, parsley, turnip greens, oranges and other citrus fruits, and certain berries, are rich in the vitamin. A six-ounce glass of orange juice contains 90 mg, nearly twice the recommended dietary allowance. Other vegetables and fruits contain moderate amounts of vitamin C; for some populations potatoes are a principal source.

A survey carried out in 1971–1972 by the Health Resources Administration of the U.S. Department of Health, Education, and Welfare in ten representative geographical areas of the country showed that one-third of the people receive less than 45 mg of vitamin C in their diets, with only 30 percent having a daily intake greater than 100 mg and only 17 percent having one greater than 150 mg. Since that time there has been a considerable increase in the number of people taking supplementary vitamin C, but the average intake of the part of the population below the poverty level of income no doubt remains very low; in 1972 only 43 percent of these people received as much as 45 mg per day.

In 1954 and 1959 Dr. W. J. McCormick, a Canadian physician, formulated the hypothesis that cancer is a collagen disease, secondary to a deficiency in vitamin C. He recognized that the generalized stromal changes of scurvy (changes in the nature of the tissues) are identical with the local stromal changes observed in the immediate vicinity of invading neoplastic cells, and surmised that the nutrient (vitamin C) that is known to be capable of preventing such generalized changes in scurvy might have similar effects in cancer. The evidence that cancer patients are almost invariably depleted of ascorbate lent support to this view.

There are some other interesting associations between scurvy and cancer. There is no real modern evidence that frankly scorbutic patients succumb to cancer, presumably because they either die fairly rapidly from their extreme vitamin-deficiency state or, more likely, are promptly diagnosed and rapidly cured. The historical literature, however, contains many allusions to the increased frequency of "cancers and tumors" in scurvy victims. A typical autopsy report of James Lind (1753) contains expressions such as "all parts were so mixed up and blended together to form one mass or lump that individual organs could not be identified"—surely an 18th-century morbid anatomist's graphic description of neoplastic infiltration.

Finally, in advanced human cancer the premortal features of anemia, cachexia, extreme lassitude, hemorrhages, ulceration, susceptibility to infections, and abnormally low tissue, plasma, and leukocyte ascorbate levels, with terminal adrenal failure, are virtually identical with the premortal features of advanced human scurvy.

All of these facts support the conclusion that vitamin C is intimately involved in cancer as well as in scurvy.

ORTHOMOLECULAR MEDICINE

Drugs are powerful substances that interact with the human body or with the vectors of disease (viruses or bacteria) in such a way as to be of value in controlling disease. Many drugs have been found to be of great value. Most drugs, however, have undesirable as well as desirable effects, such that the physician prescribing the drug or the person taking the drug must weigh the good against the harm in deciding about its use or dosage. Aspirin (the chemical substance acetylsalicylic acid) is an example of a drug with moderately low toxicity and rather few harmful side effects. The ordinary aspirin tablet contains 324 mg (5 grains), and persons seeking relief from pain or other discomfort are usually advised to take a few tablets each day. The recommended dosage is sometimes as high as 30 tablets per day, as for adult rheumatoid arthritis. The fatal dose for an adult is 60 to 90 tablets. Aspirin is the most common single poison used in suicide. About 15 percent of accidental poisonings of young children are caused by aspirin. Some people show a severe sensitivity to aspirin, such that a decrease in the rate of circulation of the blood and difficulty in breathing follow the ingestion of 1 to 3 tablets. Also aspirin, like other salicylates, has the property that in concentrated solution it can attack and dissolve tissues; an aspirin tablet in the stomach may attack the stomach wall and cause the development of a bleeding ulcer.

The anticancer drugs are far more toxic than aspirin, and their side-effects, in the customary dosages, are such as to make the patient miserable during the course of his treatment. It would clearly be beneficial to find methods of treatment of cancer that do not involve such harmful side-effects. Some such methods are known; they are for the most part included in the field of orthomolecular medicine (Pauling, 1968).

Orthomolecular medicine is, as we have said, the achievement and preservation of the best health and the prevention and treatment of disease by varying the concentrations in the human body of substances that are normally present in the body and are required for health. Among these substances are the vitamins and the essential minerals; the major foods—proteins (containing the essential amino acids), fats (an important source of energy and a source of the essential fats), and carbohydrates (the major fuel for the body, providing most of the energy needed for heat, muscular work, and various biochemical reactions); and also many important substances that are manufactured in the cells of the body—the various hormones, enzymes, neurotransmitters, *p*-aminobenzoic acid, choline, cholesterol, lecithin, and others almost without number.

Thus death by general starvation, kwashiorkor (protein starvation), beriberi, scurvy, or any other deficiency disease can be averted by the intake of an adequate amount of carbohydrates, fats, proteins, thiamine, vitamin C, and other vitamins and essential minerals. To achieve the best health the rates of intake of foods should be such as to establish and maintain in the body the optimum concentrations of essential molecules, such as those of vitamin C. The word orthomolecular (from the Greek *orthos*, right, correct) means containing the right molecules in the right amounts. The right molecules are those that are required for health and the right amounts are those amounts that lead to the best health.

The use of very large amounts of vitamins in the control of disease has been called *megavitamin therapy*. Megavitamin therapy is one aspect of orthomolecular medicine. We believe that orthomolecular methods, including in particular the intake of vitamins and other important nutrients in the proper amounts, will contribute greatly to the achievement of the significant control of cancer. There is already much evidence, discussed in the following chapters, that the prophylactic and therapeutic use of vitamin C alone has value in the control of cancer. It is especially important that vitamin C, in common with many other orthomolecular substances, has extremely low toxicity and is remarkably free of harmful side-effects, even when taken in very large doses. Unlike the chemotherapeutic agents used in the treatment of cancer, it not only increases the time of survival of the patient but also leads to improvement in general health and the feeling of well-being.

EVOLUTION AND THE NEED FOR VITAMIN C

A few years ago it began to be recognized that there is something special about vitamin C, something that differentiates it from all the other vitamins and other essential nutrients. This something is the very large difference between the optimum intake, which leads to the best health and the greatest protection against disease, and the usually recommended intake, which for most people suffices to prevent the corresponding deficiency disease, scurvy in the case of vitamin C. Thus for thiamine, vitamin B1, the daily allowance recommended by the Food and Nutrition Board of the U.S. National Academy of Sciences and National Research Council to prevent beriberi is 1.5 mg, and the optimum intake for most people may be 7.5 mg, only five times as great (it is in fact not reliably known). For most other vitamins, too, the available evidence indicates that the optimum intake is around five or perhaps ten times the recommended dietary allowance (the RDA). For vitamin C, however, the optimum daily intake for most people is probably 100 or 200 times the RDA.

It is a striking fact that all species of animals require vitamin B1 in their diets, in order to live, whereas all species of plants manufacture this substance, thiamine, in their own cells. Since animals may have evolved from plants, we may ask what the circumstances were that caused animals to lose the ability to synthesize thiamine. The primeval animal, the ancestor of all species of animals, had without doubt inherited from its plant ancestors the genes that control the production of the enzymes involved in synthesizing thiamine from its precursor molecules. The biochemical requirements of this primeval animal were, however, nearly the same as those of its immediate plant ancestors. Accordingly the animal by eating these plants was introducing into its own body essentially the amount of thiamine required for good health, and it had little need for the machinery involved in making thiamine. In the course of time a mutant appeared that had lost the thiamine-synthesis genes. This mutant was not burdened with the unnecessary machinery, and it won out in the competition with the earlier type for existence. Since then all animals, descendants of this primeval animal, have required exogenous thiamine for life.

In the same way the primeval animal lost the ability to synthesize riboflavin (vitamin B2), pyridoxine (vitamin B6), niacin (the pellagra-preventing vitamin), vitamin A, and most other vitamins.

We know, however, that this early loss of a synthetic ability did not occur for vitamin C. In fact, almost all species of animals have continued to synthesize ascorbic acid up to the present time. The horse, the cow, the dog, the cat, the sheep, the goat, the mouse, the rat—all these species and many more manufacture ascorbic acid in the cells of their bodies. Only a few animal species—man and the other primates, the guinea pig, a fruit-eating bat, the red-vented bulbul, trout and other fishes in that family (Salmonidae), some species of grasshoppers—have had the misfortune to lose this ability, so that their life and health depend upon finding food that provides a sufficient supply of this essential nutrient.

We may ask why most species of animals have continued to manufacture vitamin C. Why did not the primeval animal, who gave up the manufacture of thiamine, riboflavin, pyridoxine, niacin, vitamin A and other vitamins, not also give up the synthesis of ascorbic acid?

We know that animals differ from plants in that they make large amounts of collagen, which serves as their principal structural macro-molecule (in place of the cellulose of plants), and that ascorbic acid is required for the synthesis of collagen. Accordingly the need of animals for ascorbic acid is greater than the need of plants for this substance, and in consequence the supply in the plant-food diet would not suffice to fill the need of the animals, and a mutant animal who was unable to synthesize ascorbic acid would be at a pronounced disadvantage, such that the mutant strain would die out.

Only if the animals of one species were living in a region, such as a warm tropical valley, where the plant foods were especially rich in this substance would the mutant win out in the evolutionary struggle. Such an event seems to have taken place a few times during the last 50 million years: once for the common ancestor of man and the other primates, once for the ancestor of the modern guinea pig, and again for the other species that now require exogenous vitamin C.

These considerations permit us to get some information about the optimum intake of vitamin C for man.

First, we may ask how much ascorbic acid is present in raw natural plant foods such as those that probably were being eaten over past millennia by species of animals that have continued to supplement their intake by manufacturing additional amounts. We checked the amounts of several vitamins present in 110 raw natural plant foods, as given in the tables in the reference book on metabolism published by the Federation of American Societies for Experimental Biology (Altman and Dittmer). When the amounts of vitamins corresponding to one day's food for an adult (the amount that provides 2,500 kilocalories of energy) are calculated, as shown in Table 14-1, it is found that for several of the vitamins the average amount is about three times the RDA. For vitamin C, however, the average amount in the plant foods is 2300 mg, which is 51 times the RDA, set at 45 mg per day by the Food and Nutrition Board. This fact also indicates strongly that there is something strange about vitamin C.

If the need for vitamin C were really as small as the 45 mg per day recommended by the Food and Nutrition Board the various species of animals living on plant foods, which provide far larger amounts of this substance, would surely have given up the burden of manufacturing extra amounts of the substance in their own cells. We may accordingly conclude that 2,300 mg per day is less than the optimum intake.

The average amount of vitamin C in a day's ration of eight foods with the highest content is 12,000 mg. The ancestor of man and the other primates who lost the ability to synthesize ascorbic acid was probably living in a tropical valley where these and similar high-C foods provided this large amount of the vitamin. The other primates have for the most part continued to live in tropical

TABLE 14-1
Vitamin content of 110 raw natural plant foods referred to the amount giving 2,500 kilocalories of food energy

Foods	Thiamine	Riboflavin	Niacin	Ascorbic acid
Nuts and grains (11)	3.2 mg	1.5 mg	27 mg	0 mg
Fruit, low C (21)	1.9	2.0	19	600
Beans and peas (15)	7.5	4.7	34	1,000
Berries, low C (8)	1.7	2.0	15	1,200
Vegetables, low C (25)	5.0	5.9	39	1,200
Intermediate-C foods (16)	7.8	9.8	77	3,400
High-C foods (6)	8.1	19.6	58	6,000
Very high-C foods (8)	6.1	9.0	68	12,000
Averages for 110 foods	5.0	5.4	41	2,300
Recommended daily allowance for male adult	1.5 mg	1.6 mg	18 mg	45 mg
Ratio of plant food average to average recommended allowance	3.3	3.4	2.3	51

Nuts and grains: almonds, filberts, macadamia nuts, peanuts, barley, brown rice, whole grain rice, sesame seeds, sunflower seeds, wheat, wild rice.

Fruit (low in vitamin C, less than 2,500 mg): apples, apricots, avocadoes, bananas, cherries (sour red, sweet), coconut, dates, figs, grapefruit, grapes, kumquats, mangoes, nectarines, peaches, pears, pineapple, plums, crabapples, honeydew melon, watermelon.

Beans and peas: broad beans (immature seeds, mature seeds), cowpeas (immature seeds, mature seeds), lima beans (immature seeds, mature seeds), mung beans (seeds, sprouts), peas (edible pod, green mature seeds), snapbeans (green, yellow), soybeans (immature seeds, mature seeds, sprouts).

Berries (low C, less than 2,500 mg): blackberries, blueberries, cranberries, loganberries, raspberries, currants (red), gooseberries, tangerines.

Vegetables (low C, less than 2,500 mg): bamboo shoots, beets, carrots, celeriac root, celery, corn, cucumber, dandelion greens, egg-plant, garlic cloves, horseradish, lettuce, okra, onions (young, mature), parsnips, potatoes, pumpkins, rhubarb, rutabagas, squash (summer, winter), sweet potatoes, green tomatoes, yams.

Intermediate-C foods (2,500 to 4,900 mg): artichokes, asparagus, beet greens, cantaloupe, chicory greens, chinese cabbage, fennel, lemons, limes, oranges, radishes, spinach, zucchini, strawberries, swiss chard, ripe tomatoes.

High-C foods (5,000 to 7,900 mg): brussels sprouts, cabbage, cauliflower, chives, collards, mustard greens.

Very high-C foods (8,000 to 16,500 mg): broccoli spears, black currants, kale, parsley, hot chili peppers (green, red), sweet peppers (green, red).

areas where their food has a high content of vitamin C, but human beings have spread into other areas and their intake of vitamin C has decreased to such an extent as to cause the health of nearly every person to suffer. The biochemist Irwin Stone in his scientific papers and his book *The Healing Factor, Vitamin C Against Disease* has emphasized that essentially all human beings have been suffering from the genetic disease hypoascorbemia, a deficiency of ascorbate in the blood. This disease can be controlled only by the ingestion of the proper amount of vitamin C, which is indicated by the foregoing argument to lie between 2,300 and 12,000 mg per day.

This argument receives strong support from the studies that have been made of the amounts of ascorbic acid that are synthesized by animals of various species. Thus a goat the size of a man (weighing 70 kilograms, 154 pounds) synthesizes 13,000 mg of this vitamin each day. For other species—mouse, rat, cat, dog, cow, squirrel, even the house fly—the amount synthesized is proportional to body weight, with average about 10,000 mg per day (range 2,000 to 20,000 mg per day). The only reasonable explanation of the fact that such large amounts of ascorbic acid are made by these many animal species is that smaller amounts would lead to poorer health. Man resembles other animals so closely in his biochemistry that we may conclude that he has a similar need for this important substance.

Additional evidence is provided by the fact that the foods recommended for monkeys and guinea pigs provide about 4,000 mg of vitamin C per day, calculated to 70 kilograms of body weight.

There have been many observations by physicians and scientists that a high intake of vitamin C provides a significant amount of protection against various infectious diseases, both viral and bacterial, and also against cancer. There is now little doubt that both the incidence and the outcome of cancer are closely related to the intake of this important substance.

15

Vitamin C
and the Immune
System

It is now becoming rather generally accepted that the immune system in human beings plays a significant part in their resistance to cancer, both in the prophylactic sense of an efficient immunosurveillance system that destroys cancerous growths at an early stage in their careers and in the protective sense of retarding the growth of established malignant tumors. Patients who, because of an organ transplant or some other reason, have been maintained for a long time on a regime that suppresses their immune systems have an increased incidence of certain kinds of cancer. Moreover, cancer patients tend to have decreased immunocompetence, as measured by the standard tests. Any practical measure that would enhance immunocompetence would be beneficial both in decreasing the incidence of cancer and in helping to control the disease in the cancer patient. The treatment of cancer by immunotherapy has been discussed in Chapter 9, where brief mention was made of vitamin C in relation to immunocompetence. In this chapter we shall discuss this subject in greater detail.

The immunological defense system has the difficult task of distinguishing foe from friend by first recognizing "not-self" (the invading vectors of disease, such as bacteria, or malignant cells) as distinct from "self" (the normal cells). Recognition depends upon the evaluation of differences in molecular structure. For the viral and bacterial vectors of disease these differences are striking and their recognition is relatively easily accomplished, whereas for the cancer cells the differences are slight and the immune mechanisms must be highly competent in order to be effective.

Lewis Thomas, President of the Memorial Sloan-Kettering Cancer Center, has pictured the immune system as a police force, constantly patrolling the body and checking the cells, keeping an eye open for cells that have become malignant, and, when they have been recognized, destroying them.

There is much evidence that vitamin C is essential for the efficient working of the immune system. The mechanisms of the immune system involve both certain molecules, mainly protein molecules, that are present in solution in the body fluids, and certain cells.

The immunoglobulins are these protein molecules, often called *antibodies* or *antitoxins,* that have the power of recognizing "not-self" cells and combining with them, thus helping to mark them for destruction. It has been found that human beings with a high intake of vitamin C manufacture more antibody molecules (those of types IgG and IgM) than those with a lower intake; this work was done by Vallance (1977), who studied subjects who for nearly a year were isolated in a remote British research station in Antarctica and were in this way kept from contact with any sources of new infection (which by stimulating immunoglobulin production would have introduced a disturbing factor). The same result of increase in antibody production associated with an increase in intake of vitamin C has been observed also with guinea pigs by our colleague Dr. George Feigen.

There is another complex of protein molecules, called *complement,* that is involved in an essential way in the process of destruction of foreign cells and malignant cells, and it has been shown by Feigen that in guinea pigs an increased intake of vitamin C significantly increases the amount of the first component of complement, C_1 esterase, without which the whole complement cascade is inoperable and the "non-self" cells would not be destroyed. There is no doubt that vitamin C is required also in man for the synthesis of C_1 esterase, because this component of complement contains protein molecules that are similar to the molecules of collagen that are known to require vitamin C for their synthesis.

After the foreign cells or malignant cells have been identified and marked for destruction they are attacked and destroyed by the phagocytic (cell-eating) cells that patrol the body. The lymphocytes seem to be the most important of the phagocytic cells in the battle against cancer. A malignant tumor is often observed to be infiltrated with lymphocytes, and a high degree of lymphocyte infiltration is now accepted as a reliable indicator of a favorable outcome of the disease. Moreover, it has been demonstrated that guinea pigs maintained on very low intakes of vitamin C tolerate skin grafts from other guinea pigs, and that this tolerance is related to their abnormally low lymphocyte ascorbate levels (Kalden and Guthy, 1972). When the guinea pigs are given large amounts of vitamin C the skin grafts are promptly rejected, showing that the immune systems are again functioning. These observations and the well-known fact that leukocytes are phagocytically effective only if they contain a rather large amount of ascorbate led us to suggest in 1974 that a high intake of vitamin C would permit the lymphocyte part of the defense mechanisms against cancer to function at high efficiency. This prediction has now been confirmed. Working in the National Cancer Institute, Yonemoto and his coworkers (Yonemoto, Chretien, and Fehniger, 1976; Yonemoto, 1979) studied five healthy young men and women, 18 to 30 years old, who initially were receiving the ordinary low intake of vitamin C. They took samples of blood, separated the lymphocytes, and measured their rate of blastogenesis (production of new lymphocyte cells by budding) when stimulated by an antigenic foreign substance, phytohemagglutinin. They then gave each subject 5 g of vitamin C on each of three successive days. As is shown in Figure 15-1, the rate of formation of new lymphocytes had nearly doubled (increase 83 percent) in a few days, and it remained high for another week. A dose of 10 g per day for three days caused this rate to triple and a dose of 18 g per day caused it to reach 4 times the original value. This study leaves little doubt that a high intake of vitamin C by cancer patients increases the effectiveness of the body's protective mechanism involving lymphocytes and leads to a more favorable prognosis for the patient. More extensive studies of this sort are needed to determine the intake of vitamin C, both orally and intravenously, that leads to the maximum rate of blastogenesis of lymphocytes. The indication from the work of Yonemoto and his coworkers is that the optimum oral intake may be greater than 18 g per day.

Some very recent discoveries by Horrobin and his colleagues in Montreal have been announced just as this book goes to press. Prostaglandin E1 (PGE1) plays a major role in regulation of T-lymphocyte function, specifically increasing the body's resistance to cancer. They have discovered that the production of prostaglandin PGE1 is dependent upon dietary factors, with linoleic acid, gammalinolenic acid, zinc, pyridoxine, and vitamin C all playing key roles. Inadequate intake of any one of these will lead to inadequate PGE1 formation and thus to defective T-lymphocyte function, whereas megadoses of one are likely to be only marginally effective in this defense mechanism in the absence of adequate intakes of the others.

Another recent discovery is the finding in Massachusetts General Hospital by Dvorak and his colleagues that cancer cells tend to form cocoons of fibrin (the protein of blood clot) which protect them from immunological detection and destruction. It might be possible to counteract this mechanism for protecting cancer cells by the use of anticoagulant drugs, and indeed a number of investigators had already reported the empirical observation that the use of anticoagulants such as heparin and Warfarin exerts a beneficial retardant

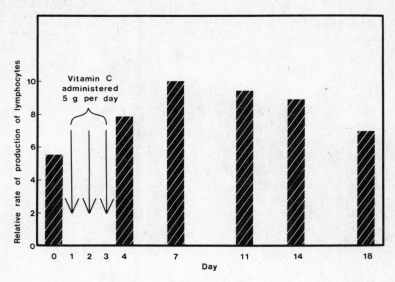

FIGURE 15-1
The rate of blastogenesis of lymphocytes (production of new lymphocytes by budding)
under stimulation by phytohemagglutinin (a plant protein used for antigenic stimulation).
The values are averages for five healthy young men or women who were given 5 g of
vitamin C by mouth on days 1, 2, and 3. (From data given by Yonemoto, 1979, averaged for
three amounts of the antigen.)

effect on both animal and human cancers. The effect of these anticoagulant
drugs would now appear to be the unmasking of the cancer cells to immunological attack.

To summarize, cancer patients generally exhibit a decreased effectiveness
of their natural immune protective mechanisms and almost invariably have a
low ascorbate content of their lymphocytes (see Chapter 17). The simplest and
safest way to enhance immunocompetence in these patients and to ensure that
their molecular and cell-mediated defense systems are working at maximum
efficiency is to increase their intake of vitamin C. Only when the increased
demand for and utilization of vitamin C in cancer are fully satisfied can these
immune mechanisms provide the maximum protection against the wayward
cancer cell.

16

Other Properties
of Vitamin C

We have emphasized in the preceding chapters the arguments that vitamin C should be effective in the prevention and treatment of cancer largely through its action in strengthening the natural protective mechanisms of the body and making them more effective. Inasmuch as these natural protective mechanisms protect us against diseases of all kinds, it is reasonable to expect that a high intake of this vitamin would have value in the prevention and treatment of these other diseases, and in fact there is much evidence that it does. Rather detailed discussions of this evidence are presented in Irwin Stone's 1972 book *The Healing Factor: Vitamin C against Disease* and in the book *Vitamin C, the Common Cold, and the Flu* (Pauling, 1976), and brief accounts are given in the following paragraphs.

VITAMIN C AND WOUND HEALING

One of the first properties of vitamin C to be recognized is that it is required for the synthesis of collagen in the human body. Collagen is the principal constituent of all connective tissue, and a good supply of vitamin C is needed whenever a healing process requires new connective tissue to be made, as in the healing of wounds, burns, and broken bones. For over forty years vitamin C has been recommended for surgical patients not only to promote healing of the surgical wounds but also to prevent surgical shock. Thus Crandon in 1955 stated that "Ascorbic acid is the only nutrient lack of which has been proved to delay or prevent wound healing in man. . . . There is evidence of an increased demand for the vitamin postoperatively. . . . Because of its ample availability and rapid absorption by all routes, there can be little excuse for surgical complications resulting from ascorbic acid lack." A representative study is that reported by Bartlett, Jones, and Ryan in 1942. A patient was scheduled to have hernia operations on both his right and his left side. The ascorbate concentration in his blood plasma was 0.9 mg per 100 ml (milliliters), indicating that he had been getting about 90 mg of vitamin C per day in his food. He was given 100 mg of vitamin C per day after the first operation, and then, some time later, 1100 mg per day after the second operation. The skin and fascia wounds on the first side healed poorly, whereas those on the second side healed well, with breaking strength three to six times that for the first side.

Forty years ago the amounts 500 mg or 1000 mg per day were recommended for surgical patients, and now much larger amounts are used by occasional surgeons. Some surgeons add 5 g of sodium ascorbate or more to each liter of intravenous fluid, in addition to giving extra vitamin C to the patient before the operation.

Extra vitamin C given to the patient undergoing an operation for cancer has, of course, the added value of helping to destroy the wandering malignant cells released into the bloodstream during the operation, thus decreasing the chance that metastases would form later on.

VITAMIN C AND THE ENCAPSULATION OF TUMORS

A closely related effect of vitamin C, resulting from its requirement for the synthesis of collagen, is that of increasing the ability of a cancer patient to encapsulate his tumor, that is, to enclose it in a membrane of scar tissue. The fortunate patient with a good supply of vitamin C may develop a very slowly growing, practically noninvasive tumor encased in a dense, almost impermeable barrier of scar tissue, giving him a clinical prognosis differing little from normal life expectancy. This encapsulation is a complex process that may involve a number of factors. One of these is always the intense local deposition of fully formed collagen fibrils that imprison the invasive tumor cells, and vitamin C is essential for this process.

VITAMIN C AND
INFECTIOUS DISEASES

Not only cancer, but also many other diseases have been reported to be controlled to some extent by an increased intake of vitamin C. The list of these diseases includes many infectious diseases, both viral and bacterial: the common cold and influenza (Pauling, 1970, 1976; Stone 1972), viral pneumonia, hepatitis, poliomyelitis, tuberculosis, measles, mumps, chicken pox, viral orchitis, viral meningitis, shingles, fever blisters and cold sores, and various bacterial infections. This property of vitamin C is especially important for cancer patients because practically all tumors ulcerate through adjacent surfaces (skin, gastrointestinal tract, respiratory tract, etc.) and become subject to secondary bacterial invasion. Efficient phagocytosis, which is dependent on a good supply of vitamin C (Chapter 15), offers some protection against this otherwise almost inevitable complication.

It is, of course, astonishing that in the last quarter of the twentieth century anyone would contend that a substance might be helpful to you no matter what disease you are suffering from. Nevertheless, the evidence is strong that vitamin C is such a substance. It is not a drug with the specific ability to fight cancer or hepatitis or any other single disease. It is instead a natural, essential substance that may participate in almost all of the chemical reactions that take place in our bodies and is required for many of them. Our bodies can fight disease effectively only when we have in our organs and body fluids enough vitamin C to enable our natural protective mechanisms to operate effectively. This amount is much larger than the amount that has been recommended by the authorities in medicine and nutrition in the past, as we have pointed out in Chapter 14.

There are very few drugs that are effective against viral infections. A natural antiviral agent is *interferon,* a protein synthesized by man and other animals that is produced by cells infected by a virus and possibly also by malignant cells and that spreads to neighboring cells and changes them in such a way as to enable them to resist infection. There is some evidence that interferon helps in the effort by the human body to control a developing cancer, and the American Cancer Society in 1979 allocated the sum of $2 million for studies of the value to cancer patients of injections of interferon. Human interferon, isolated at great expense from human blood cells, must be used, because the interferons from other animals when injected into a human being would sensitize him in such a way that further injections would cause serious allergic reactions. The suggestion that an increased intake of vitamin C would lead to the production of a larger amount of interferon (Pauling,

1970) has been verified in animals by Siegel (1974) and Schwerdt and Schwerdt (1975).

A comparison of the effectiveness against cancer and other diseases of these two orthomolecular substances, the very expensive protein human interferon and the very inexpensive nutrient vitamin C, has yet to be made.

Among the infections of special interest to cancer patients are pneumonia and viral hepatitis. A high intake of vitamin C is effective against both of these diseases. Many patients with cancer, as also many of those with other debilitating diseases, die of pneumonia. Several investigations have demonstrated the value of large doses of vitamin C in controlling pneumonia. In a recent one (Pitt and Costrini, 1979) half of a group of about 800 marine recruits in a training camp were given 2 g of vitamin C per day and the others were given a placebo. During the 8-weeks period of the trial the incidence of pneumonia was seven times as great for the placebo subjects as for the vitamin C subjects.

Serum hepatitis, involving the hepatitis-B virus, can be a serious problem for surgical patients who receive blood transfusions. In most hospitals the incidence of postoperative serum hepatitis is now kept low by the careful monitoring of the blood from donors and the rejection of the virus-contaminated units. In some countries, however, the incidence of hepatitis in surgical patients who receive blood transfusions is rather high, 7 to 10 percent. An extensive study of the value of vitamin C in preventing this infection was made in Torikai Hospital, Fukuoka, Japan, from 1967 to 1976 by Morishige and Murata, and reported by them in 1978. During this period there were 12 cases of hepatitis among 170 transfused patients who received little or no vitamin C (incidence 7 percent), whereas there were only 3 cases, all non-B hepatitis, among 1,367 transfused patients who received 2 g of vitamin C or more per day (incidence 0.2 percent). Most patients in that hospital are now routinely given 10 g of vitamin C per day.

VITAMIN C AND
CHEDIAK-HIGASHI DISEASE

Patients with the recessive genetic disease called Chediak-Higashi disease suffer frequent and severe pyogenic (pus-forming) infections that result from the abnormal functioning of polymorphonuclear leukocytes, and they also have an abnormally high susceptibility to cancer. In 1976 it was reported by a number of investigators that treatment of the patients with moderately high doses of ascorbic acid restores the bactericidal activity of the leukocytes, thus protecting them against infections, although it does not correct the abnormal morphology of the cells (references are given by Rausch et al., 1978). This clear example of the value of vitamin C against infectious diseases for these patients emphasizes its importance for the immune system in general.

VITAMIN C AND HEART DISEASE

Cardiovascular disease, disease of the heart and blood vessels, constitutes the principal cause of death. During recent years it has been discovered that nutritional and environmental factors are important in determining the incidence of cardiovascular disease. Some epidemiological evidence, such as that reported by Chope and Breslow in 1955, indicates that vitamin C is the most important of these factors.

Cigarette smoking is very harmful to the heart. The mortality rate from cardiovascular disease at each age is twice as great for cigarette smokers as for non-smokers.

Damage by oxidation is done to the unsaturated fatty substances present in the membranes of the cells in the walls of blood vessels and other tissue. These important substances are protected against this damage by vitamin C and vitamin E, which are the natural antioxidants.

Cholesterol is another natural substance with important functions in the human body. Human beings manufacture about 1000 mg per day, and in addition obtain some in their food. Some observations around 30 years ago seemed to indicate that the age-specific incidence of cardiovascular disease might be greater for people with a high concentration of cholesterol in the blood than for those with a low concentration, and now for 30 years both the American Heart Association and government agencies have made vigorous efforts to get the American people to decrease their intake of eggs and animal fat, principal sources of dietary cholesterol. Many studies of the effect of such a diet have been made, with equivocal results—it is clear that the large benefit that was expected is not observed. More thorough studies of the relation of blood cholesterol to heart disease have revealed that the incidence of heart disease has a negative correlation with the amount of high-density lipoprotein cholesterol and a positive correlation with the amount of low-density lipoprotein cholesterol in the blood; that is, high-density lipoprotein cholesterol is beneficial and low-density lipoprotein cholesterol is harmful. The factors that determine the ratio of high-density to low-density lipoprotein cholesterol are not known, except for one important one: a high level of vitamin C increases the amount of high-density and decreases the amount of low-density lipoprotein cholesterol. Both of these changes help to protect against cardiovascular disease.

VITAMIN C AS A DETOXIFYING AGENT

It is likely that part of the effectiveness of vitamin C in helping to decrease the incidence of cancer results from its power to act as a rather general detoxifying agent. In collaboration with molecular oxygen and certain enzymes in the human body, it converts toxic substances, including those that cause cancer, into nontoxic derivatives that then are eliminated in the urine. This detoxifying action has been demonstrated for scores of substances (references are given by Cameron, Pauling, and Leibovitz, 1979). Among these substances are the carcinogenic hydrocarbons, the nitrosamines, and other cancer-producing chemicals.

THE REBOUND EFFECT

When a person regularly ingests about 150 mg of vitamin C per day the ascorbate concentration in the blood plasma is about 1.5 mg per 100 milliliters. It was observed in 1973 (Harris, Robinson, and Pauling; Spero and Anderson) that when the amount ingested is increased to several grams per day the plasma ascorbate concentration rises to about 2.5 mg per 100 milliliters and then, with the same high intake, decreases over a few days to about the original value, 1.5.

This phenomenon is well known in bacteria. It is called induced enzyme formation. In the case of vitamin C in human beings, we assume that there are enzymes that help to convert ascorbate to certain oxidation products. It is known that these oxidation products serve a useful purpose—they have been shown to have anticancer activity in mice, and presumably are similarly effective in human beings. The ascorbate itself also is valuable, and accordingly on a low intake the body manufactures only a small number of the enzyme molecules, in order to conserve the ascorbate. When the high intake is begun more enzyme molecules are manufactured, in order to convert the extra ascorbate to the useful oxidation products, instead of simply allowing the excess to be excreted in the urine. These oxidation products, which as yet have not been thoroughly studied, may provide an important part of the mechanism by which large doses of vitamin C help to control cancer and other diseases.

From the foregoing argument we would expect that when a person who has been on a high intake of vitamin C for some time suddenly reverts to his original low intake the enzymes, present in large number, would operate to convert most of the ingested ascorbate to its oxidation products, leaving him with a dangerously low concentration of ascorbate in the blood. This effect has been observed; it is called the rebound effect. It lasts for only a few days, by which time the enzyme molecules present in excess have been destroyed and the number remaining has reached the value appropriate to the low intake. There is some evidence that during the period of the rebound effect the susceptibility to infections is increased; the control of cancer might also be less at this time. It is accordingly recommended that a high intake of vitamin C not be suddenly stopped, even for one day; instead it should be gradually decreased, over a period of several days, if a decrease is deemed to be necessary.

SIDE-EFFECTS OF VITAMIN C

Vitamin C is a remarkably innocuous substance, one of the least toxic substances known. Studies with guinea pigs showed that they could be given doses of 5 g per kilogram body weight per day orally or by subcutaneous or intravenous injection without developing symptoms of toxicity (Demole, 1934), and similar observations have been made with mice, rabbits, cats, and dogs. By extrapolation this represents a daily dose of 350 g in the adult human. Amounts of 200 g have been taken in one day by mouth by humans without serious consequences, and 100 g or more of sodium ascorbate have been given by intravenous infusion to patients with benefit rather than harm. Hundreds of people have taken 10 to 20 g per day over periods of years or decades with no indication of harmful long-term side-effects. The fact that animals of most species synthesize corresponding amounts (Chapter 14) makes this degree of tolerance of the substance reasonable.

There has been much discussion in newspaper articles about the possibility that a high intake of vitamin C may cause the development of kidney stones. This suggestion is largely based on a misunderstanding. It is known that some kinds of kidney stones (the less common ones) tend to form in acidic urine, and others tend to form in alkaline urine. Physicians sometimes recommend to certain patients that they keep their urine either alkaline or acidic, in case that it is known that the patient may develop kidney stones of one kind or the other. Large doses of vitamin C as sodium ascorbate keep the urine alkaline, whereas large doses of this vitamin as ascorbic acid make it acidic. This question really has nothing to do with vitamin C, because any other alkalizing agent, such as potassium citrate, can be used to make the urine alkaline, and any acidifier, such as ammonium chloride, can be used to make it acidic. Some people, of rare genotypes, such as those who convert most of the ascorbate to oxalate, may be unable to tolerate large doses of vitamin C, but the very small number of the cases reported in the medical literature indicates that there are not very many of these unfortunate individuals. The risk of kidney stone formation as a result of high ascorbate intake is very remote indeed.

A few years ago many people were disturbed and some of them stopped taking supplementary vitamin C when a report was published and widely discussed in newspapers that a high intake of vitamin C taken with a meal might destroy as much as 95 percent of the vitamin B12 contained in the food, possibly leading to a serious disease resembling pernicious anemia. Later careful studies by two groups of investigators showed that this report was erroneous, largely because a poor method of analysis for vitamin B12 had been used. The form of vitamin B12 found in foods, hydroxycobalamin, is to some extent susceptible to attack by vitamin C. In the stomachs of persons other than those with pernicious anemia, however, the B12 combines with intrinsic factor to form a complex that can be transported into the blood stream. This complex is stable: it is not destroyed by vitamin C. Moreover, the form of vitamin B12 that is present in vitamin tablets is cyanocobalamin, which is not destroyed by vitamin C. The concern about vitamin C in relation to vitamin B12 was accordingly not based on solid facts.

The most common side-effect of large doses of vitamin C is looseness of the bowels, which in some people may be described as a mild temporary diarrhea, and an increased tendency to produce intestinal gas. A few grams of vitamin C taken without other food may serve as an excellent laxative, and for cancer patients (as well as others) it may take the place of Max Gerson's enemas (Chapter 10) in clearing from the lower bowel the toxic waste material that could be harmful to the health if retained for longer times. Some people tolerate sodium ascorbate better than ascorbic acid, and tablets, including timed-release tablets, better than the pure crystalline vitamin. Most people can take 15 or 20 g per day, in divided doses (3 or more per day) without much gastrointestinal distress, and sick people can take much larger amounts.

Some practical information about vitamin C is given in Appendix IV.

17

The Utilization
of Vitamin C
by Cancer Patients

It was reported more than forty years ago that the concentration of ascorbate in the blood of cancer patients is abnormally low (Appelbaum, 1937). This observation has been verified in many later studies. At first it was assumed that such reports merely reflected the reduced dietary intake of the patients, and when these studies had been made on patients with far advanced cancer this was undoubtedly a major factor. However, as the studies have been extended to include earlier stages of cancer and patients with good appetites, it is now recognized that the low vitamin C status of cancer patients indicates an increased requirement and utilization of this essential nutrient because of the cancer. In addition it has been recognized that there is also an increased requirement and utilization of vitamin C in response to the stress inflicted on the body by conventional anticancer treatment regimes.

It is a fundamental principle of medicine to facilitate homeostasis, the tendency of the physiological system to maintain internal stability through the coordinated response of its parts to any situation or stimulus tending to disturb its normal condition or function. Sometimes the process of homeostasis occurs naturally, without the need for intervention by the patient or the physician. For example, it is important to keep the concentration of sodium ion in the blood and other body fluids constant, at the normal value. This goal is achieved by the elimination of a smaller or larger amount of salt in the urine. Sometimes, however, there is nothing that the body itself can do to regain its normal condition. Any vitamin deficiency is an example; our bodies are not able to manufacture vitamins, and accordingly a vitamin deficiency, no matter what its cause, can be corrected only by our providing a proper supply of the vitamin. As we have pointed out in Chapter 14, there is a close relation between cancer and scurvy, and there is no doubt that an essential part of the battle against cancer is to rectify the bodily deficiency in vitamin C that is caused by the cancer.

HOW WE HANDLE VITAMIN C

Under ordinary circumstances the vitamin C in the human body comes from the food that is eaten. The average intake of this vitamin by people in the United States is probably now (1979) about 100 mg per day. Most of the ingested vitamin is transferred across the intestinal wall into the blood stream, producing an ascorbate concentration in the blood plasma of about 1.0 mg per 100 ml. Essentially all of the ascorbate is converted into other substances, and there is evidence that these other substances are important in maintaining good health, even though we do not yet know very much about them and their actions. With this ordinary intake of vitamin C essentially none is lost in the urine.

THE ACTION OF THE KIDNEY

A primary function of the kidney is to remove unwanted substances from the blood. The two human kidneys contain about 2 million filtering units, called nephrons. An important part of each nephron is its glomerule or glomerular filter, which consists of a small blood vessel coiled inside a collecting bag. The blood vessel has holes in its walls to permit water molecules and other small molecules to pass through, but not the blood cells or the very large molecules of the blood proteins (serum albumin, serum globulins). The dilute urine collected in the collecting bag then passes along a long narrow tube, called a tubule, and special pumps in the walls of the tubules pump part of the water back into the blood, leaving the rest of the water, together with un-wanted small molecules such as those of urea and other waste products, to pass into the bladder and be eliminated as urine.

Some of the small molecules, such as those of sugar (glucose) and the vitamins, are, however, needed by the body. They are returned to the body by special pumps. The pump for vitamin C works nearly perfectly in conserving this vitamin up to the limit of its capacity, which is at about the plasma ascorbate concentration 1.5 mg per 100 ml, corresponding to a daily intake of about 150 mg.

If more than 150 mg of vitamin C is taken per day, some of it is lost in the urine. In most books on nutrition the statement is made that this fact shows that the body is getting rid of the extra vitamin C, and that accordingly nobody needs to take more than 150 mg per day. We believe that this argument is false. Instead, we ask why the ascorbate pump should have been developed with this large a capacity, unless it is important to conserve at least this amount of the vitamin. Our conclusion is that this intake represents a lower limit to the optimum intake.

In fact, only a fraction of the ingested vitamin C is lost in the urine—about 25 percent for a dose of 1000 or 2000 mg. The rest is retained in the body and put to good use.

TESTING FOR ASCORBATE STATUS

A rough indication of the vitamin C status of a person can be made by estimating the vitamin C content of the urine. This urine test can now be carried out very simply and cleanly using "C-Stix", manufactured by Ames Laboratories of Elkhart, Indiana and its international affiliates. This simple test not only indicates whether vitamin C is present or absent from the urine sample, but also gives an approximate measure of its concentration.

In states of vitamin C deficiency, such as in the average cancer patient, no vitamin C will be detectable in the urine. In contrast, healthy individuals maintaining a reasonable dietary intake should show some measurable urinary vitamin C concentration.

A more accurate assessment of the vitamin C status can be made by the use of a simple technique known as an ascorbic acid loading test. The person under investigation swallows a drink of juice containing a measured amount of vitamin C, usually 1 gram. The urine is then collected during the next four or six hours, and analyzed for ascorbate. The amount found for most persons is about 20 percent of the amount ingested, but ill people, especially those with schizophrenia and those with cancer, may eliminate very little. Chronic schizophrenics may have to ingest as much as 25 g or even 100 g in a day before an appreciable amount appears in the urine. There is still uncertainty about the meaning of this fact, but one possibility is that these persons manufacture a very large amount of the enzyme that helps convert ascorbate to its oxidation products, so that very little ascorbate is left in the blood. This abnormality might be responsible for their tendency to schizophrenia.

A somewhat similar observation has been made about one cancer patient. In studies of ordinary persons who had been deprived of all vitamin C for several months, bringing them to the verge of scurvy, it has been found that the intake of 2 to 4 grams is enough to replenish the tissues to such an extent that some of the vitamin appears in the urine. When Dr. Edward Greer's cancer patient (A', Chapter 21), who had been ingesting large doses of vitamin C, was taken off the vitamin for a few days it was found that an intake of 50 grams was needed before ascorbate appeared in the urine. This illustrates the rebound effect.

More accurate assessments of the vitamin C status of a person can be made by measuring the ascorbate concentration in the blood plasma and in the white blood cells.

The measurement of plasma ascorbate concentration is a relatively simple procedure that is routinely performed in most competent biochemical laboratories. The values are expressed in milligrams of ascorbate per 100 ml plasma. Normal values—that is, the values found in healthy individuals who partake of a reasonably adequate diet—average around 1 mg ascorbate per 100 ml plasma. In contrast, the usual values found in cancer patients tend to be in the 0.1 to 0.4 mg per 100 ml plasma range. The steady state level for plasma ascorbate concentration is around 1.4 to 1.5 mg per 100 ml plasma in the great majority of individuals irrespective of vitamin C intake above 150 mg per day, as discussed in an earlier section.

As one might expect, plasma levels of ascorbate represent a fluctuating pool increased by intestinal absorption and depleted in a dynamic fashion by cellular and tissue requirements. A more accurate estimation of the true vitamin C status of a person can be obtained by measuring the slower change in the vitamin C concentration in the white blood cells (leukocyte ascorbic acid), taken as representative of the body-wide concentration of ascorbate. Measurement of white-blood-cell ascorbate is a much more difficult technique and is not usually performed in most hospital laboratories. The results are expressed as micrograms of ascorbate per 100 million white blood cells (μg ascorbate/10^8 wbc).

A study of this sort is being carried out by one of us (E.C.) and his collaborators in Vale of Leven Hospital, and an interesting pattern of results is emerging.

Normal values—that is, the values found in healthy individuals—depend upon their dietary habits. Obviously higher levels are found in individuals whose diet contains a high proportion of ascorbate-rich foods such as fruit and vegetables, whereas lower levels are found in those whose diet contains smaller amounts of these ingredients.

Our studies have been concerned principally with trying to determine the requirements and utilization of ascorbate in cancer patients. For "normal" individuals we studied the spouses of our cancer patients, on the reasonable assumption that the spouses would have approximately the same age and the same social and nutritional background. To determine the effects of surgery, we also carried out leukocyte ascorbic acid assays on a few healthy patients entering the hospital for surgery with simple mechanical complaints such as a hernia.

As expected because of individual variation in dietary patterns, the results in healthy persons were spread over quite a wide range, with a few such apparently healthy individuals having remarkably low white-blood-cell ascorbate levels. The average value in over 100 such individuals, however, is around 32 $\mu g/10^8$ wbc.

In contrast, the average value in cancer patients in the same area is around 18 μg per 10^8 wbc. Furthermore, the more extensive the cancer, the lower are the available body stores of ascorbate. Thus the average value in ten women with breast cancer apparently still confined to the breast was found to be 19 $\mu g/10^8$ wbc, whereas the average value in eight breast cancer patients with known metastases had dropped to 11 $\mu g/10^8$ wbc.

If surgery is then performed on these cancer patients (or on the non-cancerous "healthy" controls mentioned above) a further significant drop in leukocyte ascorbate levels is observed. And if we subject these patients to high-energy radiation as part of their treatment for cancer the values will drop even further. For instance, we might have a breast-cancer patient starting at 20, dropping to 12 after mastectomy, and then dropping to 8 during and immediately after her course of post-operative radiotherapy. And if that patient then receives a course of anticancer chemotherapy the values will drop still lower, to 2 or 3 $\mu g/10^8$ wbc (see Figure 17-1).

Therefore as a result of the cancer and in response to anticancer treatments we have created a situation of fairly severe ascorbic acid deficiency. This interferes with the healing processes and with the body's immune resistance not only to cancer but against any intercurrent infection, and contributes to complications and the overall debility of the "cancer-plus-treatment" illness.

Because ascorbate is required for the proper functioning of so many essential biological processes, no physician should disagree that such an ascorbate deficit should be corrected. Where disagreement still exists is in regard to the quantity of vitamin C that is required to rectify this deficit. It will be recalled from the earlier discussion in this chapter that not all ingested ascorbic acid is absorbed, and that not all ascorbic acid is retained, and the greater the dose ingested the wider will become the gap between actual intake and effective absorption and utilization. Nevertheless the only way to rectify the deficit is to ensure that an adequate surplus of ascorbic acid is available at all times.

Most of our studies have been carried out on daily intakes of 10 grams, usually given in the form of sodium ascorbate, and usually ingested in four equal doses of 2.5 g spread throughout the day. We asked the healthy spouses

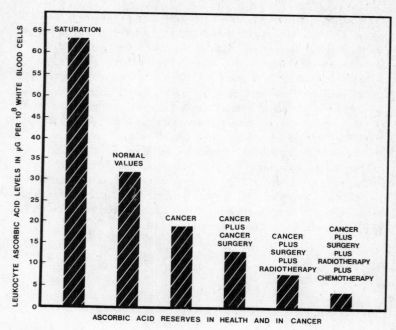

FIGURE 17-1

Values of the concentration of ascorbate in white blood cells, in micrograms per 100 million cells, for different people. The value for "saturation" corresponds for well persons to an intake of 150 mg or more per day, and the "normal values" to an intake of about 50 mg per day.

of our cancer patients to cooperate in this study and ran into an immediate problem. If healthy people not previously conditioned by taking supplemental ascorbate are suddenly placed on such a high-intake regime, few can tolerate it. As a result of ingesting 10 g of vitamin C a day, some of these healthy individuals developed heartburn, flatulence, nausea, and especially diarrhea and were forced to withdraw from the experimental study. However, many volunteers persisted, and we found that in these healthy individuals a daily intake of 10 g will bring the white-cell ascorbate level up to around the 60 to 70 range within about two weeks at most. This 60 to 70 range seems to mark saturation levels; it cannot be exceeded by increasing intake or by prolonging intake.

The cancer patients show a completely different pattern. First, almost without exception the cancer patients can ingest 10 grams of ascorbate per day without any gastrointestinal side effects. On daily intakes of 10 grams of ascorbate per day for many months, few if any reach white-cell ascorbate levels of 40 or above, and no cancer patient that we have studied has ever reached anything approaching saturation levels. Thus on a daily intake of 10 grams the depleted cancer patient can be restored to just above the range found in healthy individuals in the same population but cannot be saturated. From this information it may well be that in patients with cancer, intakes much greater than 10 g a day are necessary to obtain maximum therapeutic benefit. At this juncture we do not know the correct dose in cancer patients. Until we learn more, there is something to be said for the simple recommendation that the cancer patient should ingest each day just as much ascorbate as he can tolerate without producing troublesome gastrointestinal side effects.

The fraction of a large oral dose that is transferred across the intestinal wall into the blood stream may be less than 50 percent. Accordingly intravenous ascorbate may be more than twice as effective as oral ascorbate. Some clinical observations about intravenous ascorbate are discussed in Chapter 20.

PART IV

THE USE OF
VITAMIN C
IN THE TREATMENT
AND PREVENTION
OF CANCER

18

The Principal Trial of Vitamin C in Vale of Leven Hospital

In 1971 we reached the conclusion, on the basis of two separate arguments, that an increased intake of vitamin C should be of value in controlling cancer. One of these arguments (Cameron and Rotman, 1972) is that this increased intake would stimulate the production in the cells of the human body of the substance that inhibits the enzyme hyaluronidase, which is released by malignant tumors and which attacks the hyaluronic acid in the intercellular cement of the surrounding tissues, thus weakening these tissues and permitting their infiltration by the growing tumor. The other argument is that an increased intake of vitamin C would lead to the synthesis of more collagen fibrils in the intercellular cement, which would strengthen it and help the normal tissues to prevent the cancer from growing. These arguments seemed to us to justify the carrying out of a trial of vitamin C with patients with advanced cancer, especially since vitamin C is a constituent of foods, required by every human being for life, and is noteworthy for its very low toxicity and freedom from any serious side effects, even when taken in very large amounts.

Nevertheless, it must be recorded that the immediate reaction of one of us (Ewan Cameron) to this idea was sheer incredulity. It seemed quite ludicrous to suggest that this simple, cheap, harmless powder, which could be bought in any drugstore, could possibly have any value against such a bafflingly complex and resistant disease as cancer. But the solid logic of the arguments persisted. The ideas continued to make sense, together with the general idea that a high intake of vitamin C might make all of the body's natural protective mechanisms more effective; and the cancer patients continued to die, day after day. In such a "nothing-to-lose" situation it seemed worth a try. If the vitamin C did the patient no good, at least it would do him no harm.

CHAPTER 18

A cautious start was made in November 1971. Vitamin C (as sodium ascorbate) in what at that time seemed very high dosage (10 g per day, as was suggested by the arguments presented in earlier chapters of this book) was given to a small number of patients with very advanced cancer who were under the care of one of us (E. C.) in Vale of Leven Hospital, Loch Lomondside, Scotland. If one dares to use the word "lucky" in such a dismal situation, we were indeed lucky in the chance that selected these first few patients. They responded very dramatically indeed, being converted from a hopeless, terminal, "dying" situation into a hopeful "recovering" situation. It was a very exciting start—it seemed almost too good to be true.

But then after some time the first few ascorbate-treated patients died, and some of the newer patients did not respond so dramatically to the ascorbate treatment, so that we passed through a period of real self doubt. Were we achieving anything? Were we deluding ourselves? Worse still, although we had not published any report at that time, were we in danger of deluding others and raising unjustified hopes? Fortunately, we continued to prescribe ascorbate for our dying cancer patients and also, with increasing confidence, for many other cancer patients at much earlier stages in their illness. Now, eight years and many hundreds of cancer patients later, we are in a position to make a cautious assessment of its worth.

Vitamin C is not a miraculous cure for cancer, but it goes a long way toward the therapeutic goal outlined in Chapter 4. It significantly prolongs the life of the cancer patient. Moreover, it improves the condition of the patient to such an extent that his life during his remaining months or years is comfortable, contented, useful, productive, and satisfying. Because of the low cost of vitamin C and the decreased need for special care, the financial burden of the treatment to the patient and his family is small. We believe that supplemental ascorbate can be of real help to all cancer patients and of quite dramatic benefit to a fortunate few.

It is now recognized that cytotoxic chemotherapy has for the most part failed to live up to its earlier promise, at least so far as the common, solid, well-differentiated malignancies of adult life are concerned, and there is a growing awareness among both patients and their physicians that treatments with these toximolecular substances may be just as unpleasant and just as lethal as the disease that they are prescribed to treat. During the past twenty-five years, the period when aggressive cytotoxic chemotherapy has become the vogue, the survival rates for the majority of human cancers have shown no improvement. There is now a desperate search under way for some alternative mode of treatment. We believe that the deliberate enhancement of the body's natural mechanisms of resistance to cancer offers a promising way out of the present impasse, and that the provision of supplemental vitamin C is at the present time the most promising way of attaining that aim.

Vitamin C, as ascorbic acid or sodium ascorbate, can be taken alongside all conventional forms of cancer therapy—before and after surgery, during and after radiotherapy, together with hormones when hormone therapy is indicated, together with immunostimulants, and together with cytotoxic chemotherapy, although, as is discussed later, there is without doubt significant interaction of ascorbate and the various chemotherapeutic agents, about which we still have little detailed knowledge.

Many cancer patients reach a stage when it is clear that the conventional forms of treatment no longer are effective. It is with patients of this sort that the most clear-cut evidence about the value of vitamin C against cancer has been obtained. In the eight years of the Vale of Leven studies essentially all of the first 500 patients to receive ascorbate were in the terminal, "untreatable" state; that is, for them and for hundreds of other cancer patients in the same hospital the possible value of conventional therapy had been exhausted. Except that vitamin C was given to some of them, these patients received no treatment except routine nursing care and morphine or diamorphine as needed to control pain. Through the comparison of the ascorbate-treated "untreatable" patients and the similar "untreatable" patients who received the same medical care except for no ascorbate, a real assessment of the benefit of the ascorbate could be made.

Subjective benefit, improvement in the feeling of well-being expressed by the patient, is hard to measure scientifically, but it is still the objective of all good doctoring. Giving vitamin C in large dosage to patients with advanced cancer produces subjective benefit in almost every patient by about the fifth day. The patient will claim to feel better, stronger, and mentally more alert. Distressing symptoms such as bone pain from skeletal metastases diminish and may even disappear completely. Objective evidence of improvement is also observed. The patient becomes more lively and shows more interest, and also eats more food, indicating that he has a better appetite and is no longer feeling nauseated and miserable.

In Chapter 10 we talked about the placebo effect and the observer-anticipation effect, saying that if any treatment, even a carefully measured dose of distilled water, is given with conviction to cancer patients, a fraction of the patients will swear that they have benefited, and their therapists, if they sincerely believe in the regime, will be equally convinced that some degree of benefit has accrued. We are well aware that some placebo effect might have operated in the Vale of Leven studies, but we are convinced that it has played only a small part. Moreover, there is also a reverse psychological effect.

Dying cancer patients, having endured the whole gamut of conventional anti-cancer therapies and seen them fail, may wish to grasp at straws, but deep in their hearts they know these straws to be unsubstantial, and in particular they are hardly likely to be fooled by vitamin C, with all of its "health-food, vitamin-quack" connotations. Indeed, it was hard for us to believe that this familiar substance, vitamin C, could possibly do much good. But it did do good, and even the most skeptical and experienced observers were before long convinced of its value. No matter what the mechanisms of its action might be, there soon was no doubt that when dying cancer patients were given large doses of vitamin C they felt much better—and that is one of the most important objectives of good medical care.

In the first Vale of Leven clinical publication on vitamin C and cancer (Cameron and Baird, 1973) there was described the quite dramatic relief of bone pain in four out of five patients with expanding skeletal metastases, and the view was advanced that this beneficial effect resulted from retardation of invasive growth of the tumors in their inelastic environment. The striking observation was also made that these patients, who had been receiving large doses of morphine or diamorphine, did not show any of the usual withdrawal signs when the narcotic drug was discontinued and did not complain of with-drawal symptoms. This observation was the basis for the use of large doses of vitamin C in the treatment of narcotics addiction (Libby and Stone, 1977).

In the next clinical report (1974) Cameron and Campbell described the first 50 patients with advanced cancer who received 10 g of vitamin C or more per day. It was expected that most of these patients (90 percent) would die within about three months; in fact, only half of them had died on or before the 100th day after being deemed to be "untreatable," at which time the administration of ascorbate was begun. The others lived much longer than expected. Twenty of them died after from 110 to 659 days, average survival time 261 days, and five were still living when the report was written (10 July 1974), with average survival time greater than 610 days. Even though no formal comparison with patients who did not receive the vitamin was made, it seemed certain that the ascorbate-treated patients were living much longer than would have been expected.

Of equal importance was the observation that most of the ascorbate-treated patients entered a period of increased well-being and general clinical improve-ment. The benefits enjoyed by a majority of these patients included, in addi-tion to increased well-being, relief from pain, a decrease in malignant ascites and malignant pleural effusions, relief from hematuria, some reversal of malignant hepatomegaly and malignant jaundice, and decrease in the red-cell sedimentation rate and in the serum seromucoid level, all accepted indicators of lessening malignant activity. It was thus possible to conclude that both the increase in well-being and the apparent increase in survival time resulted from a significant attack by the ascorbate, either directly or by way of the natural protective mechanisms of the body, on the malignancy itself.

Our next task was to get more reliable information about the magnitude of the increase in survival time of the ascorbate-treated patients. The generally accepted way of getting this information is to carry out a double-blind randomized clinical trial. Hundreds of these trials, involving tens of thousands of patients with advanced cancer, have been carried out in order to test various conventional therapies, especially the use of various combinations of anticancer drugs. Patients entering such a trial are randomly allocated to one or the other of two groups, with those in one group receiving the substance under test and those in the other group receiving similar tablets containing some inactive substance, and with neither the patients nor the doctors and nurses conducting the trial knowing which patients are receiving the active substance and which are receiving the placebo, this information being kept by some other person, not directly involved in the study, until the trial is over and the progress of the patients has been assessed. Sometimes the patients are in matched pairs (matched as to age, sex, type and stage of disease, etc.), with one of each pair, selected by toss of a coin, given tablets of one kind and the other given those of the other kind.

We have not been able to carry out such a double-blind randomized clinical trial of vitamin C in relation to advanced cancer, for several reasons.

In 1971, when the work with vitamin C began in Vale of Leven Hospital, we did not have enough information about vitamin C and cancer to plan such a trial. We did not know what the effect of a large intake of this vitamin, 200 times the usual intake, on the cancerous growth would be—there was the chance that it would be catastrophic. The vitamin was accordingly administered to the first few patients with great caution, and they were carefully watched for signs of harmful effects. It then became evident that the patients were not being harmed by the vitamin, but were receiving benefit, and the time came when enough knowledge had been accumulated to permit a double-blind randomized clinical trial to be planned. By that time, however, Ewan Cameron had become so convinced of the value of large doses of vitamin C to patients with advanced cancer that he was unwilling for ethical reasons to withhold it from any patient to whom he had the power to give it; accordingly he could not carry out such a trial with his patients.

We then strove to arrange that other investigators, who had not reached this position, should carry out controlled trials. In the spring of 1973 one of us (Linus Pauling) went to Bethesda, Maryland, to show several officers of the U.S. National Cancer Institute the case histories of Cameron's first 40 ascorbate-treated patients and to ask that the National Cancer Institute carry out a controlled trial. The suggestion was rejected. We continued to make this recommendation to the National Cancer Institute, year after year, until finally, in 1978, Dr. Vincent DeVita, the officer of the NCI in charge of clinical trials, arranged that such a trial be carried out under the direction of Dr. Charles Moertel of the Mayo Clinic (see Chapter 19).

We also made preliminary arrangements with other investigators, in Scotland and Japan, to carry out double-blind randomized trials of vitamin C in patients with advanced cancer, if money to support the work could be obtained, and we applied to the National Cancer Institute for a grant for this purpose and related work. The application was rejected by the National Cancer Institute and also by the American Cancer Society.

We have heard, however, that there are several other clinical trials now under way without the support of the NCI or the ACS, and the results should be available within a year or two.

Even though we could not carry out a double-blind randomized clinical trial, we could carry out a controlled trial. The Vale of Leven Hospital is a large hospital, with 440 beds, and it registers about 500 new cancer patients each year. Although Dr. Cameron was the Senior Consultant Surgeon in administrative charge of the 100 surgical beds, he was in direct medical charge of only some of these cancer patients. At first none of the other physicians or surgeons gave large doses of vitamin C to their patients, and even in later years many of the Vale of Leven cancer patients have not received this treatment. Thus there have been other cancer patients closely similar to the ascorbate-treated patients, receiving the same treatment, except for the ascorbate, from the same medical and surgical staff, in the same hospital, and these patients can serve as the controls.

In 1976 we reported the survival times of 100 terminal cancer patients given supplemental ascorbate and those of a control group of 1,000 patients of similar initial status treated by the same clinicians in the same hospital, and who had been managed identically except for the supplemental ascorbate. The 1,000 controls consisted of 10 control patients for each ascorbate-treated patient, matched as to sex, age, primary tumor type, and clinical status of "untreatability." We employed an outside doctor, who had no knowledge of the survival times of the ascorbate-treated patients, to examine the case histories of each of the 1,000 control patients and to record for each of them the survival time—the time in days between the date of abandonment of all conventional forms of treatment and the date of death.

The results were surprising, even to us (see Figure 18-1). On 10 August 1976 all of the 1,000 control patients had died, whereas 18 of the 100 ascorbate-treated patients were still living. On that date the average time of survival after the date of "untreatability" was 4.2 times as great for the ascorbate-

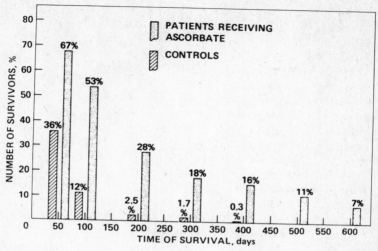

FIGURE 18-1

The percentage of 1000 controls (matched cancer patients) and the 100 patients treated with ascorbic acid (other treatment identical) who survived by the indicated number of days after being deemed "untreatable." The values at 200, 300, 400, 500, and 600 days are minimum values corresponding to the date August 10, 1979, when 5% of these patients (and none of the controls) were still alive.

treated patients as for their matched controls. By 15 May 1978 eleven more of the ascorbate-treated patients had died, and the survival-time ratio had increased to 5.6. Five of the seven others continue to live 16 months later, and this ratio is now 6.6 (on 15 September 1979). The 100 ascorbate-treated patients have lived on the average about 300 days longer than their matched controls, and in addition it is our strong clinical impression that they have lived happier lives during this terminal period. Moreover, five of them continue to survive, still taking their daily doses of sodium ascorbate, and some of them might well be considered to have been "cured" of their malignant disease, in that they are free of overt manifestations of cancer and are leading normal lives.

We considered this to be a remarkable achievement, bearing in mind that if the mortality of cancer could be decreased by 5 percent the lives of 20,000 American cancer patients would be saved each year.

Because of the importance of the problem of cancer, we made a second study of the Vale of Leven patients in 1978, again with 100 ascorbate-treated patients and 1,000 matched controls. Ten of the original 100 ascorbate-treated patients, mainly with rare forms of cancer for whom it had been difficult to

TABLE 18-1

Differences in average survival times of ascorbate-treated patients and matched controls

| Primary tumor type | Patients, no. | | Mean survival times, days | | | | Increased survival times of ascorbate-treated patients, days* | | |
| | Test | Controls | From first hospital attendance | | From date of untreatability | | E | F | G |
			A Test	B Control	C Test	D Control	A–B	C–D	
Colon	17	170	458+	316	352+	33	142+	319+	324
Bronchus	17	170	219+	118	186+	31	101+	155+	184+
Stomach	13	130	286+	159	182+	32	127+	150+	134+
Breast	11	110	1396+	1020	487+	52	376+	435+	378+
Kidney	8	80	774+	492	381+	39	282+	342+	348+
Bladder	7	70	1669+	420	355+	21	1249+	334+	226+
Rectum	7	70	634	336	270	43	298	227	247
Ovary	6	60	884	366	183	69	518	114	157
Others	14	140	706+	279	278+	37	427+	241+	189+
All	100	1000	681+	360	293+	38	321+	255+	234+

*E, calculated as A – B; F, calculated as C – D; G, additional survival time of first set of ascorbate-treated patients with first set of controls, ref.(1) to 15 May 1978, when seven of them were still living (measured from the date of untreatability). The + following a number indicates that one patient in the group (two in the bladder group) continued to survive after 15 May 1978.

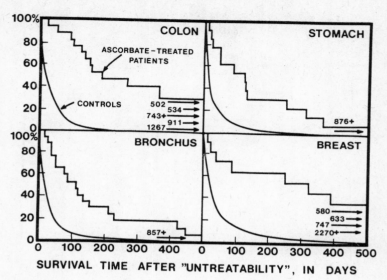

FIGURE 18-2

Percentage of survivors at times after date of onset of terminal stage (untreatability) of ascorbate-treated patients with primary cancer of colon, stomach, bronchus, or breast, compared with that for matched controls (10 per ascorbate-treated patient).

find sets of exactly matched controls, were replaced by new ones, and the 1,000 matched controls were independently selected, without regard as to whether or not they had been selected before (about half of them were in the earlier set). The results of this study are given in Table 18-1 and Figures 18-2 and 18-3. The 100 ascorbate-treated patients and their matched controls (same type of primary tumor, same sex, and same age to within five years) are divided into nine groups, based on the type of primary tumor; for example, 17 ascorbate-treated patients and 170 controls with cancer of the colon. The mean survival times were measured from the date of first attendance at hospital with cancer and also from the date when the patient was determined to be "untreatable"; that is, when the conventional therapies were deemed to be no longer effective—it was at this date or a few days later that ascorbate treatment was begun.

Column E in Table 18-1 gives the difference in average survival time of the ascorbate-treated patients and that of the controls; that is, it gives the average increase in survival time of the ascorbate-treated patients relative to the controls, measured from the date of first hospital attendance. Column F gives the average increase in survival time measured from the date of "untreatability."

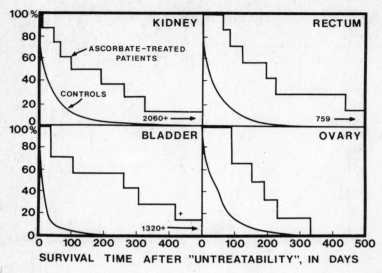

FIGURE 18-3
Percentage of survivors at times after date of onset of terminal stage (untreatability) of ascorbate-treated patients with primary cancer of kidney, rectum, bladder, or ovary, compared with that for matched controls (10 per ascorbate-treated patient).

Column G gives the same quantity, as determined in the 1976 study, brought up to the later date (15 May 1978).

The numbers in the three columns differ somewhat from one another, but the differences are those to be expected from the large range of values for the individual patients. The most striking fact is that every value is positive; that is, in each of the nine cancer categories (colon, bronchus, etc.) and each of the three tests (E, F, G) the ascorbate-treated patients on the average lived much longer than their matched controls.

Although the matched controls were selected without consideration of the date of death or whether death had occurred, none was still living at the time when Table 18-1 was compiled. The explanation of this fact is that cancer patients who reach a terminal stage have a life expectancy of only a few months at most. Nevertheless, it seems worthwhile to compare the controls with the 92 ascorbate-treated patients who had also died when Table 18-1 was prepared, measuring survival time in both groups from the date of first hospital attendance to the date of death, the two reference dates that are exactly known. This comparison gives 251 days as the increase in average survival time of the ascorbate-treated subjects over the value for the controls, compared to 321 + days when all 100 ascorbate-treated subjects and their controls are included.

Of the 1,000 control patients, 370 were completely concurrent with the ascorbate-treated patients. The mean value of the survival times of these completely concurrent control patients was 327 days measured from the date of first hospital attendance and 42 days measured from the date of untreatability, compared with 379 and 36 days, respectively, for the overlapping and historical controls. The values of the increase in survival time of the ascorbate-treated patients over that for the completely concurrent controls are 354 + days (from date of first hospital attendance) and 257 + days (from date of untreatability); the average is 306 + days. These values, with use of the 370 completely concurrent controls, are a little larger than those with use of all 1,000 controls (average 288 + days for the two reference dates). The average of the values for the concurrent controls and all controls, equally weighted, is 297 + days.

From all of these considerations we reached the conclusion in 1978 that there is strong evidence that treatment of patients in Scotland with terminal (untreatable) cancer with 10 g of vitamin C per day increases their survival time by an average of 300 + days (as of 15 May 1978). The sign " + " indicates that some of the ascorbate-treated patients were still alive at that time—8 out of 100. Of these 8, 5 are alive 16 months later, and the increase in mean survival has now reached 330 + days (15 September 1979).

There is little doubt now that a high intake of vitamin C is beneficial to most patients with advanced cancer. The beneficial effects seem to apply to all kinds of cancer, but we are quite unable to predict the degree of benefit likely to occur in any individual patient. Therapeutic responses to vitamin C in patients with advanced cancer range from dramatic regressions to no measurable benefit whatsoever, with the majority of patients occupying an intermediate category of benefit sustained for a significant period of time, but with eventual death from the original disease or some intercurrent illness.

It is our conclusion that this simple and safe treatment, the ingestion of large amounts of vitamin C, is of definite value in the treatment of patients with advanced cancer. Although the evidence is as yet not so strong, we believe that vitamin C has even greater value for the treatment of cancer patients with the disease in earlier stages and also for the prevention of cancer.

19

Other Clinical Trials

A few other clinical trials of vitamin C with cancer patients have been carried out, as described in the following paragraphs.

EARLY TRIALS

The first report of clinical benefit to cancer patients from moderately large doses of ascorbate is that of the German physician W. G. Deucher in 1940. He verified that patients with advanced cancer had a low body concentration of ascorbate (Chapter 17), and claimed that a regime of 1 to 4 g of ascorbate each day for several days had a remarkably good effect on the general state of health of the patients and on their ability to withstand heavy doses of high-energy radiation; in some patients the improvement was so great as to be "very astonishing" to the physicians in direct charge of the patients. A number of similar reports were then published in the German medical journals, with all of the physicians agreeing that administration of ascorbate (usually 1 or 2 g per day, together with some vitamin A) to cancer patients coincided with an improvement in well-being and occasionally in tumor regression. (References to these early reports are given by Stone, 1973, and by Cameron and Pauling, 1979.) On consideration of these favorable observations between 1940 and 1960 it is hard to understand why studies of the use of vitamin C in the management of cancer comparable in extent and thoroughness to those carried out during the last 25 years for the cytotoxic anticancer drugs have yet to be made. The National Cancer Institute, the American Cancer Society, and the

American Medical Association seem long ago to have accepted the false idea that the only value of vitamin C is to prevent death by scurvy, that only a few milligrams per day are needed for this purpose, and that larger amounts could not possibly be effective in controlling any disease—surely not such a ravaging and difficult-to-control disease as cancer.

Only one of the early reports, that by the American physician Dr. Edward Greer in 1954, dealt with the use of large doses of vitamin C over a period as long as 18 months. Greer's remarkable patient (A') is discussed in Chapter 21. A more recent study by Cheraskin and his associates (1968) describes a synergistic effect of supplemental ascorbate on the radiation response in patients with squamous-cell carcinomas of the uterine cervix. Twenty-seven patients were given 750 mg of ascorbic acid per day, beginning one week before the radiation treatment and continuing until three weeks after its termination; in addition they received a vitamin-mineral supplement and general nutritional advice (decrease in intake of sucrose). The controls were 27 similar patients who did not receive the vitamins or nutritional advice. Radiation therapy was equally vigorous for the two groups. The response to the radiation was significantly higher for the nutritionally treated patients (average score 97.5) than for the controls (average score 63.3). Thus there is some evidence that cancer patients undergoing radiotherapy have an increased requirement for ascorbic acid, and that satisfying this increased requirement protects against some of the harmful effects of irradiation as well as potentiating the therapeutic response.

THE FUKUOKA TORIKAI HOSPITAL STUDY

In 1979 Morishige and Murata published a report on all the patients with apparently terminal cancer who had been admitted to the Fukuoka Torikai Hospital, Fukuoka, Japan, with the diagnosis of cancer during the five year period 1 January 1973 to 31 December 1977. The fraction of cancer patients receiving large doses of vitamin C had increased steadily during this period. Of the 99 patients with apparently terminal cancer 44 received 4 g of vitamin C or less per day and 55 received 5 g or more per day. The average times of survival after the date when the patient was designated as terminal (average 10 days after admission to the hospital) are shown in Table 19-1 and Figure 19-1. The death rate of the low-ascorbate patients was about three times that for the high-ascorbate patients, as was found also in the Vale of Leven study. None of the low-ascorbate patients survived more than 174 days, whereas 18 (33

TABLE 19-1
Average survival times after date of designation as terminal of Fukuoka Torikai cancer patients receiving varying amount of vitamin C

Location of primary tumor	Amount of vitamin C (grams per day)			
	0–4	5–9	10–29	30–60
Stomach	41 (17)*	124 (3)	115 (5)	90 (9)
Lung	50 (6)	91 (3)	100 (1)	54 (5)
Uterus	44 (4)	601 + (3)	780 + (2)	243 + (3)
Others	43 (17)	281 + (5)	276 + (5)	164 + (11)
All	43 (44)	275 + (14)	278 + (13)	129 + (28)

* The numbers of patients in each group are given in parentheses.

percent) of the high-ascorbate patients survived longer than 174 days, their average (on 10 August 1978) being 483 days. Six of the high-ascorbate patients were still alive when the report was written, with average survival 866 days.

We see from Table 19-1 that the effect of 5 to 9 g of ascorbate per day is about the same as that of 10 to 29 g per day, and that 30 to 60 g per day had a smaller effect. Morishige and Murata say, however, that there is the possibility that this apparent decreased effectiveness of the largest doses resulted from their use with patients with the poorest prognosis.

Morishige and Murata also report that, in agreement with the observations of Cameron and Campbell (1974), in many patients the administration of vitamin C seems to improve the state of well-being, as indicated by better appetite, increased mental alertness, and desire to return to ordinary life.

THE MAYO CLINIC TRIAL

A carefully designed double-blind trial of the value of vitamin C in comparison with a placebo has been carried out in 1978–79 (Creagan, Moertel, O'Fallon, Schutt, O'Connell, Rubin, and Frytak, 1979). This study was designed to repeat the Vale of Leven study, but there was one important difference. Cytotoxic chemotherapy is used in Scotland only rarely in the treatment of adult patients with solid tumors, and only four of the 100 ascorbate-treated patients in the Vale of Leven study had received courses of chemotherapy. On the other hand, 52 of the 60 ascorbate-treated patients in the Mayo Clinic study had received courses of chemotherapy before the study was begun, as had also 56 of the 63 patients in the placebo group. It is known that cytotoxic chemotherapy damages the immune system and might prevent the vitamin C

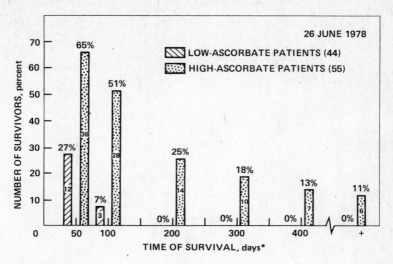

FIGURE 19-1

The percentages of the 44 low-ascorbate terminal cancer patients (4 g per day or less) and of the 55 high-ascorbate terminal cancer patients (5 g per day or more, average 29 g per day) in Fukuoka Torikai Hospital who survived by the indicated number of days after being deemed terminal. The six high-ascorbate patients still alive had on August 10, 1978 lived an average of 866 days after the apparently terminal date (Morishige and Murata).

from being effective, inasmuch as it functions mainly by potentiating this system (Chapter 15). In the Mayo Clinic study the investigators reported that they were unable to demonstrate any statistically significant benefit of vitamin C, 10 g per day, greater than that of the placebo. The fraction of patients who claimed some improvement in symptoms during the treatment was 58 percent for the placebo group and 63 percent for the ascorbate-treated group, and the median survival times after the start of the study were 6 weeks and 8 weeks, respectively.

The Mayo Clinic investigators conclude their paper with the statement that they "cannot recommend the use of high-dose vitamin C in patients with advanced cancer who have previously received irradiation or chemotherapy." We do not agree with this conclusion. Comparison of the results of the Vale of Leven study and the Mayo Clinic study shows that previous courses of chemotherapy interfere with the beneficial action of vitamin C. However, the Mayo Clinic ascorbate-treated patients seem, from the report by Creagan *et al.*, to have received some benefit from their vitamin C, as is mentioned above. Since treatment with vitamin C involves no danger and little expense, it is hard for us to understand why the patients with advanced cancer who have gone through treatment with cytotoxic chemotherapy should be deprived of the benefit of vitamin C, even though this benefit would have been greater if they had not been subjected to chemotherapy.

The relation of vitamin C therapy to high-energy radiation and chemotherapy is discussed further in Chapter 23.

THE VALE OF LEVEN
LUNG-CANCER STUDY

In order to get some additional information about the value of vitamin C in comparison with other methods of treating patients with advanced cancer, a study was made of the survival times of all patients with lung cancer who were admitted to Vale of Leven Hospital between 23 November 1971 and 22 November 1976.

Vale of Leven is a District General Hospital without a specialized thoracic-surgery service. In addition, the District of some 120,000 people is served by separate out-patient clinics specializing in respiratory diseases. As a result, most patients with lung cancer are referred elsewhere, and those admitted to Vale of Leven Hospital tend to be suffering from advanced incurable disease. During the 5-year period that was studied only one patient of the 126 admitted with lung cancer was found to be suitable for curative treatment, in his case surgery. This patient is still alive, five years after his treatment by lobectomy.

Of the remaining 125 patients, 14 were treated with high-energy radiation, 17 with chemotherapy (Mustine or Cyclophosphamide), and 24 with ascorbate; 70 received no treatment other than narcotics to control pain. The average survival times after the date of first hospital attendance with illness (bronchial carcinoma) recognized to be incurable are, for the four methods of treatment, 184, 90, 187 +, and 68 days, respectively. One of the ascorbate-treated patients is still alive on 15 September 1979, with survival time 1346 days.

The patients who received radiotherapy or chemotherapy may initially have had a slightly better prognosis than the others, but we believe that the selection of patient between ascorbate-treated and no-treatment was essentially at random—the chance assignment to one or another unit in the hospital.

The patients selected for treatment by radiotherapy enjoyed a significant increase in survival time, average 184 days as compared to 68 days for the untreated patients. The average survival time of the patients treated with chemotherapy, 90 days, is only marginally greater than that of the untreated patients, whereas that for the ascorbate-treated patients, 187 + days, is significantly greater.

COLONIC POLYPOSIS
AND COLORECTAL CANCER

Colonic polyposis is a genetic disease characterized by the formation of large numbers of polyps in the colon and rectum. These polyps are benign tumors but their presence has long been recognized as a pre-malignant condition. According to Willis (1973), "Victims of familial polyposis are almost certain to die of carcinoma of the colon or rectum at an early age." There is, however, now hope for them. Studies by DeCosse et al. (1975), Lai et al. (1977), and Watne et al. (1977) with 16 persons with familial polyposis gave the result that the regular intake of 3 g of vitamin C per day caused the polyps to disappear in half of the patients. There is a real possibility that a larger intake, of 10 or 20 g per day, would control the disease in others.

CONCLUSION

Only a few clinical trials of the effectiveness of vitamin C have been carried out. Many such trials are now needed to determine the proper dosages and the relation of vitamin C to conventional treatments as well as to other nutritional regimes.

20

Case Histories of Vale of Leven Patients

In this chapter we give accounts of the progress of a number of patients with advanced cancer who were treated with large doses of vitamin C in Vale of Leven Hospital, and also of three other cancer patients in a nearby hospital. Some of the Vale of Leven patients have been included because they responded especially well but others have been selected to represent less successful responses to ascorbate treatment.

Case A (ovarian carcinoma)

Mrs. A, age 68, one of our very first patients, was operated upon in October 1971 and found to have inoperable ovarian carcinoma with large tumor masses occupying the whole pelvis and extensive tumor deposits throughout the peritoneal cavity. The cytotoxic agent Thio-Tepa was instilled once intraperitoneally more as a tradition than in any expectation that it would do any good. Mrs. A went home to die, but had to be readmitted toward the end of November because of distressing malignant ascites (the accumulation of fluid within the abdominal cavity). This fluid was drained, and the large tumor masses could be easily palpated. She was commenced on an intravenous infusion of sodium ascorbate solution, 5 grams per day for 7 days, then the same amount by mouth, and improved dramatically. She became mentally more alert, her appetite returned, and she became ambulant. What seemed to us unbelievable was that the large tumor masses steadily shrank in size and eventually became impalpable. Then quite suddenly one Sunday evening, about four weeks after ascorbic acid had been commenced, she became rapidly very ill indeed, vomiting profusely and with profound circulatory collapse, and she died a few hours later. Her survival time was only 33 days. An autopsy was performed, and the findings were almost unbelievable. The very large tumor masses had disappeared, although small nodules of tumor were still present scattered here and there throughout the abdominal cavity. Many soft fibrous adhesions had formed, and the actual cause of death was high intestinal obstruction from these adhesions. Examination of sections of the small residual tumor nodules showed that the tumor was still actively dividing, and yet the great bulk of tumor tissue had disappeared. It seemed likely that all tumor would eventually have disappeared completely, had death from an intercurrent complication not intervened.

Although her survival was so brief, she remains one of our most remarkable patients. Unfortunately in the great majority the tumor does not disappear as a result of ascorbate treatment. Instead, the patient appears to enter a standstill phase during which the tumor neither advances nor regresses, and this standstill phase may persist for appreciable periods of time, during which the patient may enjoy a return to comparative well-being and good health. But because cancer progression is such a complex situation, with many other factors influencing the outcome, the response of individual patients may vary widely on either side of this average response.

Terminal cancer is a complex situation, with progress of the disease at any time depending upon the delicate balance reached between tumor-growth-promoting factors on the one hand and the various host defensive factors on the other, and with the overall trend always toward accelerating tumor dominance. If one could introduce into this complex equilibrium a single further factor capable of enhancing host defense in a safe and physiological way, one could logically predict a whole spectrum of therapeutic responses, which might be classified in the following way:

1. No response (or at least a therapeutic response so slight as to be unrecordable)

2. Minimal response

3. Retardation of tumor growth

4. Cytostasis (or "standstill effect")

5. Tumor regression

6. Tumor hemorrhage and necrosis

We present records of patients who occupy each of these categories.

GROUP 1: NO RESPONSE

By "no response" we mean that there was no definite evidence that ascorbic acid had caused any real tumor retardation, but even in this, the lowest, category many patients claimed to have enjoyed at least some subjective evidence of benefit. They said that they felt better. It might be considered unnecessary to describe a typical "no response" patient, but we intend to do so just to show how difficult it is to evaluate such clinical and human problems, and to decide whether or not any benefit has accrued.

Case B (ovarian carcinoma)

Mrs. B was a slim attractive suburban housewife, age 49, married to a prosperous naval architect. They had no family. In May 1969 a total hysterectomy and bilateral salpingo-oopherectomy (removal of the whole womb and both ovaries and fallopian tubes) had been carried out for an ovarian cancer, which at the time of surgery seemed quite localized and favorable. She returned to hospital in January 1972, losing weight and rather miserable. She had quite gross liver enlargement from multiple liver metastases, confirmed by radio-isotope liver scan. She was started on ascorbate (10 g per day, orally) and continued as an outpatient attending review clinics once per month. During this time she was able to continue running her home, doing her shopping and even some light gardening. Both she and her devoted husband were well aware of the diagnosis and the ultimate prognosis, and also understandably skeptical about the value of vitamin C. In spite of these obstacles, however, both did claim that she felt somewhat better and stronger as the weeks went by. There was no really convincing evidence of this, and the size of her liver remained unchanged. Then fairly suddenly in August, seven months after commencing ascorbate, her condition deteriorated very rapidly, with deepening jaundice, ascites (free fluid in the abdominal cavity), and the sudden appearance of multiple lung metastases. She died from her cancer 226 days after starting her ascorbate.

It is tempting to consider the intervening seven-month period as a standstill effect caused by ascorbate therapy, but a "gain" of seven months in an illness that had already lasted nearly three years has to remain of doubtful significance.

GROUP 2: MINIMAL RESPONSE

In the category of minimal response we include patients who obtained definite and striking benefit, but with the benefit short-lived. Three patients will serve to illustrate this situation.

Case C (breast cancer)

Mrs. C was a plump jolly widow of 53 with a grown-up family, who had all left home. She first attended Vale of Leven Hospital in May 1970 with a breast cancer that at first appeared to be localized. Within weeks after surgery, however, she complained of backache, and investigations showed metastases in the lumbar vertebrae. She was treated by palliative radiation to the spine, with excellent symptomatic relief, and then by an appropriate hormone regime, but with only transient, if any, benefit. By June 1971 she had developed extensive malignant recurrence in the armpit and the neck. Further radiotherapy was given and the hormonal regime was changed, but it was quite clear that this was a losing battle. On 10 December 1971 she was brought to the hospital by ambulance to die. By this time she was utterly miserable, bedridden, and in constant pain requiring heavy morphine sedation, later changed to heroin. She had extensive involvement of lymph nodes, innumerable skin metastases, and metastases in the ribs, the thoraco-lumbar spine, and the pelvis—the classical picture of far advanced cancer. She was started on ascorbate (5 g per day intravenously, then 8 g per day orally) and enjoyed a very dramatic response. By as early as the fourth day her bone pain had disappeared, and she wanted no more morphine or heroin. She became mentally alert and ambulant about the ward, and about a week later insisted that she go home and attend to her domestic affairs (she had a pet dog that would be missing her). And she did manage her own affairs, looking after her house, shopping, and no doubt comforting her pet dog, and this happy state continued for about two and a half months. One evening she collapsed suddenly at home with headache and visual disturbance, was admitted to our hospital, and died a few days later from widely disseminated cancer, 77 days after beginning ascorbate therapy. During her two and one half months' reprieve and period of comparative well-being there was no clear change in her innumerable skin and lymph-node metastases. They may not have been increasing much in size, but they certainly showed not the slightest sign of disappearing.

Case D (lung cancer)

Mrs. D was a housewife, 48 years old, with a relatively young family. She had a very gradual onset of illness toward the end of 1971 with little more than slight increase in breathlessness. This slowly progressed and became more and more disabling. She did not seek any medical advice, however, until sudden tense swelling of her face and neck brought her hurriedly to the hospital in July 1972. She had an inoperable lung cancer that had spread to the mediastinum and was literally strangling the venous drainage from her head and neck. Palliative radiotherapy was given, with relief of the venous back-pressure problems but with little or no benefit to her breathing difficulties. She continued to lose weight and to become more and more disabled, and, to complicate her situation, her husband died quite suddenly from a coronary infarction, leaving her even more emotionally crushed. She was readmitted as an emergency patient, having been found unconscious at home following an epileptic fit. Re-examination confirmed the presence of a large lung cancer, and electroencephalography indicated the presence of multiple brain metastases. At this time her life expectancy was measurable in days, or at the most a few weeks. She was started on ascorbate (10 g per day intravenously for 4 days, then orally), and within a matter of days became quite alert and rational, and with genuine improvement in her breathing problems. In contrast to the expectation on her admission, she became fit enough to go home, where she continued in a reasonably stable condition for over two months, and then rather quickly (while still taking her ascorbate, so far as we know) she developed a crop of skin metastases and died in coma a few days later, after 84 days of treatment with ascorbate.

Case E (carcinoid of appendix and cecum)

In June 1969 Mrs. E., the 69-year-old wife of a market gardener, was admitted as an emergency patient with a provisional diagnosis of acute appendicitis. At surgery the same evening, however, she was found to have a carcinoid tumor of the appendix and cecum without obvious spread. A right hemicolectomy was performed, and the prognosis was thought to be good. She continued in reasonably good health until mid-1975, when abdominal discomfort and weight loss became marked, together with a complaint of frequent hot flushes and a significantly elevated urinary level of a serotonin breakdown product (5-hydroxyindole acetic acid) that established malignant recurrence beyond doubt. In September 1975 she began to receive sodium ascorbate, 10 g per day orally, and claimed to notice an immediate improvement. Her abdominal discomfort lessened, she gained weight, and her distressing episodes of flushing became less severe and less frequent. She remained in reasonably stable condition on ascorbate with symptomatic relief for some 8 months, but by May 1976 clear signs of deterioration were present. She was admitted in July 1976 for terminal care and died a few days later from a combination of recurrent carcinoid tumor in the pelvis and liver and congestive cardiac failure.

These three patients did not live very long, but there is no doubt that they enjoyed a temporary remission of very advanced illness and a brief but quite dramatic relief of symptoms.

GROUP 3: RETARDATION
OF TUMOR GROWTH

Case F (cancer of the gallbladder)

Mr. F was a retired textile plant worker, 67 years old, who had enjoyed good health throughout his entire working life, apart from minor dyspepsia. He became ill in December 1972 with fairly sudden loss of appetite, sharp weight loss, and deepening jaundice of some three weeks' duration. At surgery he was found to have an irresectable cancer of the gallbladder. No by-pass procedure was possible, and surgery was limited to performing a confirmatory biopsy. By mid-February he was deeply jaundiced, and it seemed beyond dispute that he would have died within a few weeks from obstructive hepatic failure. He was commenced on ascorbate, 10 g per day intravenously for 9 days and then 8 g per day orally, and both subjective and objective evidence of improvement were evident within a week, with return of appetite, weight gain, and, most significantly of all, a steady clearing of his jaundice. The jaundice had cleared completely by April. He continued to take ascorbate and remained at home, if not robustly super-fit, at least moderately comfortable and active for several months. Then some signs of his illness reappeared and he died peacefully at home 205 days after starting ascorbate treatment.

Case G (stomach cancer)

Mr. G was a vigorous young oil company executive of 42 who developed stomach cancer, diagnosed on a business trip to the United States. He returned to Scotland, where a partial gastrectomy (see Chapter 5) was performed. At surgery there was no obvious evidence of tumor spread. Within a few months, however, he had developed widespread liver and intra-abdominal metastases, causing intestinal obstruction requiring further palliative by-pass surgery and during which the diagnosis was confirmed. The second operation relieved his acute symptoms, but his general condition deteriorated fairly rapidly. He was started on ascorbate (10 g per day intravenously for 5 days, then orally) and steadily improved, so much so that he was soon able to return to his rather hectic business life. He died fairly abruptly from what was assumed to be a second episode of intestinal obstruction, 258 days after commencing ascorbate in the terminal phase of his illness.

Case H (lung cancer)

Mr. H was a 31-year-old non-smoker, an ambitious business executive in a highly competitive field. He developed an irresectable cancer of the lung. A course of radiotherapy was given with little or no benefit, and his general health was deteriorating rapidly, with profound weight loss, cough with blood-stained sputum, and breathlessness on even mild exertion. He was well aware of the diagnosis, and was quite desperate, with a young family and heavy mortgage payments scheduled for years ahead. He was started on ascorbate, 10 g per day, and, perhaps because of a combination of ascorbate and sheer will-power, the transformation in this young man was remarkable. Within a few weeks he was back in business, and going out of his way to demonstrate how fit he was. This demonstration took the form of playing two consecutive rounds of golf and winning, or playing several sets of tennis in the evening after a hard day at the office. Throughout this period of clinical improvement there was no doubt that his whole life had been transformed, but there was no appreciable change in the size of his lung cancer, as shown by x-rays. Then one Saturday night, after two rounds of golf and a particularly strenuous session of squash, he collapsed, was admitted to the hospital in a drowsy confused condition, and died within a matter of days. In this man's case, his total time on ascorbate was not very long, 150 days, but there seems no doubt that progression of his cancer and of his general illness had been dramatically arrested for almost all of that period.

These three patients, typical of many more, illustrate what is perhaps the most difficult of all groups to define, the group with growth retardation. This definition has been reached on the basis of the facts that they all lived longer than had reasonably been expected, considering the extent of their disease at the onset, and, perhaps more important, that they had enjoyed a fairly dramatic improvement in their well-being during this period of intermission.

GROUP 4: CYTOSTASIS, THE STANDSTILL EFFECT

In Group 4 we include those patients in whom tumor growth appeared to have been halted for a significant period of time after the treatment with ascorbate was initiated.

Case I (pleural mesothelioma)

Mrs. I is a wealthy attractive woman in her early forties. Four years ago she was diagnosed in Memorial Sloan-Kettering Cancer Center, New York, as suffering from pleural mesothelioma, a particularly vicious form of cancer that is virtually untreatable and with usually a very short life expectancy. She started taking vitamin C, 10 g per day, on Dr. Cameron's advice, is still fit and well, and when last heard from (July 1979) was leading an archeological expedition. Her chest x-rays have remained unchanged throughout this period.

Case J (cancer of the colon)

Mr. J was a consultant engineer with an international practice. In March 1975 he developed recurrent diarrhea thought at first to be due to dysentery brought on by his frequent business visits to the Far East. Later that year the correct diagnosis of colonic cancer was established, and a sigmoid colectomy in the presence of innumerable liver metastases was performed. He was informed of the diagnosis, and began immediately post-operatively to take 10 g of sodium ascorbate per day. At the age of 48 he was somewhat older than Mr. G, but he showed the same intensity of will to overcome his illness. He continued his international consulting practice, involving frequent arduous business trips between Scotland and the United States, the Gulf Oil States, Singapore, and Australia, and in any free time in this punishing schedule he managed to indulge in his favorite pastime, ocean yacht racing, captaining his own 45-footer and winning some cups. This happy state of affairs continued throughout the whole of 1976. In February 1977 he required emergency readmission to the hospital because of acute purulent cholecystitis, and at cholecystectomy, by the same surgeon, the liver metastases were thought to be marginally larger although the patient himself remained in apparent good health. Toward the latter part of 1977 he suffered periodic feverish episodes, and biochemical indicators showed that his malignant disease was slowly progressing. Immunotherapy was added to his ascorbate regime but without benefit, and he died peacefully at home on 29 December 1977, more than two years after being totally hopeless in the conventional sense. Autopsy showed considerable fibrous stroma to the tumor, which was necrotic in places.

Case K (cancer of the colon)

Mr. K was one year older than Mr. J and he showed almost identical pathology, many liver metastases being found during the course of a palliative resection for a carcinoma of the splenic flexure of the colon. The operation was carried out on 30 December 1974, and the anastomosis was protected by a cecostomy. On the fourth post-operative day the cecostomy leaked, leading to a fecal peritonitis and endotoxic shock requiring intensive resuscitation. He recovered from this grave complication and started on ascorbate, 10 g per day orally, in mid-January 1975, at which time opacities were present on his chest x-ray photographs, virtually certainly indicating metastases in addition to the known spread to the liver. By April 1975 there was a marked reduction in the size of the presumed chest metastases, which eventually disappeared, and the patient remained robustly well. He was an intelligent man, a schoolmaster, but we are convinced that he had no idea of the true diagnosis. He soon started behaving in a somewhat eccentric manner. He lived in a small village about six miles from the hospital and joined to it by a fairly steep hill road. Instead of driving to the hospital for his follow-up visits, he first started walking and then jogging the round trip to show his fitness. This was eccentric because he had never before shown any interest in sport or physical activities. Eccentric or not, we have a picture of this middle-aged man jogging 12 miles, rain or shine, over a hill road to make his hospital visits, something his surgeon certainly could not do. This behavior continued for over 12 months, when he himself decided to stop taking his ascorbate supplements because he felt so well. He died a few weeks later in May 1976, nearly 18 months after reaching an untreatable situation.

Case L (stomach cancer)

Mrs. L is a frail, garrulous 73-year-old Irish woman who has a cancer of the stomach with large hepatic metastases. She has had this cancer now for nearly four years, during which time she has taken vitamin C, 10 g per day, and the size of the large palpable tumor has never changed. As of 15 September 1979 she had shown this standstill effect for 1364 days after the beginning of the treatment with ascorbate.

Case M (cancer of the colon)

In 1975 Mr. M, a newly retired carpenter, then aged 65, left Scotland to stay with his son in Australia. Quite soon after his arrival he developed persistent diarrhea that resisted all the usual symptomatic medications and he began to lose weight. A barium enema in Australia was "suspicious" of cancer of the sigmoid colon, and he decided to return to Scotland for treatment. There in April 1976 the diagnosis was confirmed, and a palliative sigmoid colectomy was performed in the presence of multiple metastases involving the whole liver. Soon after surgery he was started on sodium ascorbate, 10 g per day orally. He made a rapid post-operative recovery, gained weight, and became free from symptoms. Continuing on supplemental ascorbate, and remaining to all intents and purposes quite well, in July 1977 he again visited his son in Australia and stayed for about a year. Throughout the remainder of 1978 and the first half of 1979 he has had regular follow-up examinations at Vale of Leven Hospital and he still shows no clinical or biochemical evidence of any active disease. In June 1979, more than 3 years after the diagnosis of multiple liver metastases was established and on no treatment other than supplemental ascorbate, he was accepted for permanent emigration to Australia after full independent medical examination. At the time of writing (September 1979) he remains fit and well, enjoying his retirement in the Southern Hemisphere and still faithfully taking his supplemental ascorbate.

Case N (cancer of the colon)

Mrs. N, a doctor's housekeeper, then aged 56, was admitted to hospital in November 1972 with a year's history of bowel irregularity. At laparotomy performed on 27 November 1972 she was found to have a primary resectable carcinoma of the sigmoid colon and a solitary but significantly large (7.5 cm in diameter) irresectable liver metastasis. A palliative resection of the primary tumor was performed and a few days later she was started on sodium ascorbate, 10 g per day. Regular clinic attendances until December 1974 showed no evidence of any active progressive disease and she remained in apparent good health. She failed to keep her next review appointment in April 1975, having moved to stay with her daughter in another part of the country, and we subsequently learned that she died there in late May 1975, about 2½ years after starting ascorbate. Two points about this patient are of special interest. It is virtually certain that, because of her move, her ascorbate was suddenly discontinued a few weeks befor her death, coinciding with a brisk deterioration in her general condition. Also, within 48 hours of her commencing oral ascorbate she complained of sharp pain in the right upper abdomen, which was the site of the known liver metastasis (although this was not known by the patient). This discomfort was aggravated by movement but not by deep breathing and appeared to intensify soon after each oral ascorbate dose, but the whole complaint gradually subsided over a period of some five days.

Case O (ovarian cancer)

Mrs. O, the 49-year-old wife of an unemployed shipyard laborer attended the hospital for the first time in March 1973 in a terminal condition. She stated that until a few weeks before she had enjoyed good health. Her complaints were of rapidly increasing abdominal distension and rapid wasting elsewhere, nausea, anorexia, and bowel and bladder irregularity. She had a tense ascites, and 5 liters of blood-stained fluid (containing clumps of malignant cells) was removed by paracentesis (insertion of a tube through the abdominal wall). A hard craggy fixed mass some ten inches in diameter could then be easily felt in the pelvic cavity, together with malignant increase in the size of the liver, leaving no doubt as to the diagnosis of disseminated inoperable ovarian cancer. Over the next few weeks of hospitalization her ascites rapidly recurred, requiring paracentesis for relief every four to six days, some 4 to 5 liters of fluid being withdrawn on each occasion. During this time, as one would expect, there was a very rapid deterioration in her general condition, with progressive cachexia and an expectation of life measurable in weeks at most. In early May 1973 she began to receive intravenous sodium ascorbate on a dose schedule of 45 g per day continuously for 10 days, followed by 10 g per day by mouth thereafter. This high intravenous dose schedule produced some minor problems of sodium overload and fluid retention with ankle edema, which subsided completely in time. The improvement in the patient's general demeanor was quite remarkable; some four to five days after the intravenous regime was begun this almost moribund woman became ambulant and took to walking about the ward wheeling her drip-stand suspending her ascorbate infusion flask. Within some 17 days of commencing intravenous ascorbate, contrary to clinical expectation, she was judged fit enough to return home. She remained comparatively well for almost four months, with no recurrence of her ascites, but on repeated abdominal examination there was no obvious change, increase or decrease, in the size of her palpable tumor, or the degree of her malignant liver enlargement. She then voluntarily reduced her ascorbate intake, eventually to zero, mainly because of nausea but also because she had read a newspaper report denigrating its possible value. Her ascites slowly recurred, requiring further paracentesis for symptomatic relief, and she died some six months after the ascorbate regime had been initiated. We suspect, but have no way of proving, that she would have lived longer had she continued her ascorbate regime. What is beyond dispute is that her rapidly recurrent malignant ascites was completely controlled during the whole period of her ascorbate medication.

GROUP 5: TUMOR REGRESSION

We have already made mention of Mrs. A, who enjoyed a remarkable tumor regression only to die in a few weeks from complications. Other patients in this category have been more fortunate.

Case P (lymphosarcoma of the small intestine)

Mr. P is an Italian restaurateur long domiciled in Scotland. He is plump, jovial, retired, and in his early seventies. About three years ago he developed abdominal cramps, anemia, and weight loss, the cause of which was only finally diagnosed at laparotomy (an exploratory operation). He was found to have an obstructing tumor of the small intestine, with the rather unusual appearance of innumerable tiny metastases diffusely spread throughout the liver. The obstructing tumor was resected, and the unusual appearance of the liver was explained by the histology—the tumor was a lymphosarcoma. This is a relatively rare form of cancer, usually highly malignant, but also usually responsive to chemotherapeutic regimes. The palliative surgery relieved his immediate symptoms. Chemotherapy was proposed, but refused by the patient and his immediate relatives. About two months passed in comparative well-being before his health started to deteriorate, with anorexia, further weight loss, and progressive lassitude and anemia. By then he was prepared to accept chemotherapy. He was commenced on the standard MOPP regime, as described in Chapter 7. The first treatment was given with, in his case, even more than the usual unpleasant side effects; it converted an ill old man into an extremely ill old man. His leukocyte and platelet counts dropped to near-fatal levels. The second course proposed after the usual two-week interval had to be postponed for seven weeks, until his blood count returned to approximately normal levels. The second course was delivered with even more disastrous responses than the first. (To put it bluntly, it nearly killed him; but this nearly fatal iatrogenic poisoning of one person has not blinded us to the benefits of chemotherapy in certain well-defined situations.) If proof were needed, we waited another ten weeks before bringing him into hospital again with a respectable leukocyte and platelet count for his third course of chemotherapy, this time at approximately half the standard dosage. Even with this change, the side effects were rather disastrous, and we had to agree with relatives that this man was dying, not so much from his cancer as from the drugs we were using to treat him. No further chemotherapy was proposed, and he was started on ascorbate, 10 g per day. We have to report that now, three years later, Mr. P has returned to his usual jovial self, with no clinical evidence of any progressive disease. Skeptics may say that his two and a half courses of chemotherapy cured him, but we doubt this. The real practical point is that a man dying, from his disease and its treatment, is now to all intents and purposes perfectly fit and well, taking 10 g of vitamin C each day, and no other form of treatment.

Case Q (prostate cancer, lung cancer)

Mr. Q is a retired locomotive engineer in his late sixties. He has had two cancer problems to cope with. In late 1974 he became an emergency admission because of acute retention of urine superimposed upon a two-year history of progressive prostatism. Transvesical prostatectomy was performed without incident, but histology revealed prostatic adenocarcinoma. As a prophylactic measure he was commenced on stilbestrol, 5 mg per day, and he remained in apparent good health until a relatively brief illness in late 1975 led to his hospital readmission in January 1976 because of brisk weight loss, respiratory distress, and pleurodynia (rib-cage pain on inspiration). Chest x-ray photographs showed a tumor mass in the left lung, approximately 6 cm in diameter. There was nothing clinical or biochemical to suggest reactivation of his prostatic cancer. The films were regarded by consultant radiologists, physicians, surgeons, and radiotherapists to be quite diagnostic of an inoperable hilar cancer of the lung. (It has to be stressed that this is the one illustrative patient quoted in this chapter where histological proof of the diagnosis was not obtained. However, on review of the films it would be difficult to suggest any other diagnosis.) Radiotherapy and cytotoxic chemotherapy were both proposed, but in the considered judgment of the responsible clinicians it was unanimously decided that neither form of conventional treatment had anything to offer. The man was clearly dying and hopelessly incurable. He was given vitamin C at the standard dose level of 10 g a day and improved very rapidly; he was able to leave the hospital two weeks later, and within two months the sizeable lung shadow had completely disappeared. At this time (15 September 1979) this man is a happy grandfather enjoying his retirement in apparent good health, 1345 days after beginning ascorbate treatment.

Case R (cancer of the pancreas)

Mr. R. was a railroad employee in retirement. He was in his late seventies, living alone in a country cottage. He developed painless jaundice, and at surgery was found to have a fairly massive cancer of the pancreas with spread to the hilar lymph nodes. The tumor was inoperable, but it was possible to perform a by-pass procedure, allowing his bile to drain back again into his intestine; his jaundice cleared, and this period of comparative well-being lasted some eight months. But eventually his obstructive jaundice returned and he had to be readmitted into the hospital to die. He was started on vitamin C, 5 g per day orally, and, contrary to all expectation, he steadily improved. His jaundice cleared completely and he returned to his country cottage. His "eccentricity" was timber-felling and delivering the resultant firewood to one of the authors every two or three weeks. Then, some months later, something happened to him that we still cannot understand, far less explain. During the course of one weekend this active independent old man was reduced to a bizarre physical wreck and brought in by ambulance—confused, obstreperous, complaining of intense pruritus (skin itching), and with a rapidly deepening bronze pigmentation of his skin (not jaundice) and a striking steroid facies (the "moon-face" characteristic of those given large doses of steroids). He died within 48 hours, and the autopsy did not reveal the cause of death. He was found to have some bronchopneumonia but hardly to a potentially fatal extent, and his adrenal glands showed some relative thinning of the cortex (where steroids are produced) but not to a very significant extent. The only really significant finding was that he no longer had any cancer of his pancreas. His pancreas was quite small and shrivelled, and serial microscopic sections right through it showed nothing malignant, but the kind of rag-bag diagnosis of "chronic sclerosing (scarring) pancreatitis." He had survived 317 days after beginning ascorbate therapy.

Case S (cancer of the colon)

Mr. S, one of our earlier patients, had many points of similarity to Mr. R. Long before we had ever thought of vitamin C, back in 1969, this retired house painter, then 69 years old, was admitted to the hospital with sub-acute large bowel obstruction. After the usual pre-operative preparation, surgery was performed. A palliative resection of a particularly large tumor mass (an adenocarcinoma) involving both the transverse and the descending colon, the omentum, and an infiltrated loop of the small intestine was performed. There was no question of this being in any way a curative procedure, cutting through tumor tissue "en bloc," but it did relieve his immediate symptoms. Indeed, it worked better than might reasonably have been expected, because he lived for some three years thereafter, including surviving a minor cardiac infarction in the process. But then his disease caught up with him, and he also came into the hospital to die in January 1972. At that time he was the typical end-of-the-road cancer patient, sliding down life's escalator at an increasing rate with steady upper abdominal pain of increasing intensity, increasing distaste for any food, progressive weight loss, and rapidly deepening jaundice. Apart from the obvious fact that this man was dying, the striking feature of his disease was his significant degree of liver enlargement in a knobby fashion, and although in his case no secondary diagnostic laparotomy was performed, there could be no doubt about the diagnosis. He was started on vitamin C (8 to 10 g per day orally) and, to everyone's surprise, he got better. His jaundice cleared completely in a month or two, and his enlarged liver soon became impalpable. In fact, fairly rapidly this dying man returned to his previous status of a retired house painter, living quietly with his elderly wife. We mentioned some similarities with the previous patient—both men in their seventies, both dying from cancer, both jaundiced, and reversal of this process in both men, allowing them to return to their previous life. There was another point of similarity: both men were fiercely independent, this one even more so than Mr. R. Having got better, this perverse old man consistently refused to attend any of our follow-up clinics, although he insisted that his vitamin C be regularly delivered to his home, and complained bitterly on the telephone if there were even a one-day delay. One of our young research assistants had to make a round trip of 100 miles every month, to assess his state and to take routine blood samples. But, as with his predecessor on this list, something sudden and catastrophic happened to him. After more than three years on ascorbic acid, during which time this previously dying man had enjoyed good health with certainly no manifestation of active malignant disease, one Friday night he suddenly went quite berserk, threatening his wife with a meat cleaver. Police were called and within hours he was forcibly incarcerated in a State mental institution. His vitamin C was stopped, and he died there three days later. No autopsy was performed, and the cause of death was certified as being "bronchopneumonia and senile dementia." We learned of this sad episode only two weeks later. The actual cause of death is far from clear, but what remains beyond dispute is that this dying cancer patient enjoyed complete remission of his illness for three years and six months after initiation of his intake of vitamin C.

Case T (breast cancer)

Mrs. T is a pleasant housewife in her mid-fifties. About three years ago she had a mastectomy followed by radiotherapy for a centrally placed cancer of the breast. About twenty months later she developed neck pain, and x-rays showed a metastasis in the sixth cervical vertebra. She was given local radiotherapy to the affected region, with relief of pain, and commenced on the appropriate hormonal regime. Her condition continued to deteriorate and she became totally quadriplegic (paralyzed from the neck down). In addition she developed a large lytic (bone-dissolving) metastasis in the bony pelvis. She was started on ascorbate, 10 g per day, and progressively over a period of months the radiological appearance of this metastasis changed completely. It shrank in size, became calcified, and is now trabeculating; that is, the bone architecture is returning to a normal pattern. These serial x-rays cannot be interpreted in any way but as indicating regression. Unfortunately, Mrs. T remains quadriplegic from permanent compression damage to her spinal cord.

Case U (cancer of the kidney)

Mr. U presented somewhat similar features to Mrs. T. He was a 55-year-old shipyard engineer who came to the hospital with a painful swelling of his right eighth rib. He was a fit, powerfully built man actively at work. Investigation demonstrated the swelling to be an apparently solitary metastasis from a symptomless 6-cm cancer of the right kidney. The right kidney and the right eighth rib were surgically removed, and he returned to work. Within five months he returned, complaining of pain in his right shoulder and left hip, and x-rays showed lytic metastases at both these sites. At this stage this man was not dying, but he was clearly incurable by any conventional form of therapy. He was started on ascorbate, 10 g per day orally for 396 days and 20 g per day orally for 259 days, and claimed that his pain had been relieved. More significantly, serial x-rays showed the same pattern of recalcification and retrabeculation of his bone metastases. He remained well for over a year and back at work, and during this time he succeeded in reducing his golf handicap by two strokes. Then some blood tests indicated reactivation of his disease. His dose of ascorbate was doubled from 10 to 20 g per day, and the blood tests returned to normal. He continued in a reasonably static condition for another six or seven months, and then his disease dramatically reasserted itself in spite of his continuing ascorbate intake. Within a matter of weeks the beneficial changes in the known metastases reversed completely, many new metastases appeared, and after a comparatively brief terminal illness he died comatose in the hospital just under two years from starting ascorbic acid. The total survival time here was not by itself remarkable, but the serial x-ray changes clearly indicate that genuine tumor regression had occurred.

Case V (reticulum-cell sarcoma)

Mr. V, a patient of our close clinical colleague Dr. Allan Campbell of Hairmyres Hospital, Glasgow, is of special interest. The patient is a long-distance truck driver now in his late forties. He was admitted to the hospital in October 1973 as an extremely ill man. He gave a story of accelerating weight loss, extreme lassitude, excessive night sweats, pleuritic pain in the chest, and breathlessness on the least exertion. His liver and spleen were palpably enlarged, and he had numerous enlarged lymph nodes in the neck and armpit. Chest x-ray photographs showed enlargement of the mediastinum, an opacity in the root of the right lung, and a right pleural effusion. One of the enlarged neck glands was removed for microscopic examination and reported to be reticulum cell sarcoma, a very malignant form of cancer of the lymphatic system with some similarities to Hodgkin's disease, but with a poorer prognosis. Treatment of this rapidly-dividing form of malignancy by a combination of radiotherapy and chemotherapy offers a fair prospect of success, and such a course of treatment was decided upon, and his transfer to another hospital offering such facilities was requested. Because of a sudden backlog of patients requiring radiotherapy, however, he could not be transferred immediately, and he was started on intravenous ascorbate, 10 g per day. It must be stressed that this was not the first choice of treatment, but was merely planned as a holding operation for this gravely ill man until conventional treatment would be available. The response was unexpectedly dramatic: within less than two weeks all clinical manifestations of his disease had resolved, and his chest x-ray photographs rapidly returned to normal. When, somewhat belatedly, he could be accepted for radiotherapy there was nothing left to treat, so no treatment was given other than continuing his ascorbic acid, 10 g per day by mouth. This was in October 1973. Mr. V left the hospital and went back to driving his heavy articulated truck. As the winter months passed, he continued to be so fit and well that very real doubts began to be felt about the correctness of the original diagnosis. His ascorbate intake was gradually reduced, to 7½ g per day in January, 5 g per day in February, 2½ g per day in March, and none at all during April; and at the end of that month he was in trouble again, not so desperately ill as he had been originally, but sick with a recurrence of his original symptoms of lassitude and weight loss, and with a chest x-ray picture, which in the interim had been normal, showing a recurrence of his mediastinal glandular enlargement and a return of his pleural effusion. He was given 10 g per day of vitamin C by mouth, but two weeks later he was if anything worse. He was then taken back into the hospital and an intravenous regime of 20 g per day was instituted for 14 days, followed by 12.5 g per day orally. This was a very worrying period, with concern that conventional treatment was being withheld from this patient, but courage prevailed, and the patient gradually responded and eventually recovered completely. All this happened in October 1973 to June 1974, and today he remains perfectly fit and well with no evidence of any active disease, and one of the sights of Hairmyres Hospital is a massive articulated truck driving up to the hospital pharmacy once a month to collect the driver's flask of vitamin C. We should add that the slides from this patient have been examined by a panel of pathologists from both sides of the Atlantic and all agree with the original diagnosis. This patient was described in the scientific literature in 1975, and his significance is summarized in our closing paragraphs: "'Spontaneous' regression of human cancer is a rare occurrence brought about by an increase in host resistance acting through mechanisms which are virtually unknown. It could be argued that the first very dramatic remission in this patient was a 'spontaneous' regression which by pure chance coincided with the administration of ascorbic acid. However, we believe that the pattern of progressive disease up to the time of introducing treatment, *followed* by rapid remission while receiving high-dose ascorbic acid supplements, *followed* by relapse when this form of medication was withdrawn, *followed* by a further remission when this form of treatment was reinstituted, makes it virtually certain that we were observing a direct therapeutic response." In effect, this man acted as his own "off-treatment" control.

Case W (breast cancer)

Mrs. W is the wife of a prosperous company director and the mother of three children, one of whom died some years ago from leukemia. In December 1968 this patient, then 49 years old, presented in hospital with a centrally situated scirrhous adenocarcinoma of the breast with nipple retraction. A left simple mastectomy was performed, followed by a standard course of postoperative radiotherapy to the left chest wall and related lymph nodes. At that time the outlook seemed quite favorable. At follow-up examination in December 1970, however, malignant involvement of the left-armpit lymph glands was obvious. This was treated by surgical excision of all of these glands (their involvement being confirmed microscopically) and a course of hormone therapy (androgens) was instituted. By January 1971 malignant involvement of glands in the root of the neck was discovered, again confirmed by excision biopsy. Oophorectomy (see Chapter 8) was carried out in February 1972, and a microscopical examination of the excised ovaries showed that they already contained deposits of secondary breast cancer, indicating that such small metastatic deposits were already quite widely distributed as a result of blood-borne dissemination (Stage IV). Immediately after oophorectomy she was commenced on ascorbate, 10 g per day, and has been taking it without fail ever since. She remains extremely fit and well, with no clinical suspicion of any active malignant disease. A remission of advanced breast cancer after oophorectomy is enjoyed only by a minority of such patients, and in that minority a six-months remission is still considered good going. Remission of over one year is rare enough as to be somewhat remarkable. A remission lasting over seven years is, to the best of our knowledge, unknown, except for this case. We are therefore strongly convinced that credit must be given to vitamin C for this happy outcome.

GROUP 6: TUMOR
HEMORRHAGE AND NECROSIS

The reports in the sequence groups 1 to 5 have demonstrated increasing benefit to cancer patients. We have found it to be possible to go even further. In a few patients the antitumor effect is so sharp and pronounced that the overall result can be disastrous for the individual patient. Our last three illustrative case histories demonstrate a pronounced antitumor effect, and also show that ascorbate can be potentially lethal in advanced cancer and must be prescribed with caution.

Case X (reticulosis)

Mr. X, another patient of our associate Dr. Allan Campbell, was a 34-year-old insurance clerk. He was admitted to Dr. Campbell's hospital in early October 1977 with a relatively short history of lassitude, diffuse aches and pains, nocturnal sweating, low-grade fever, and weight loss of some 28 pounds in the preceding two months. Although he was clearly ill, he presented few diagnostic physical signs, and his grossly disturbed hematological and biochemical findings indicated either an acute inflammatory or an active neoplastic disorder. On the basis of one dubiously positive blood culture, a provisional diagnosis of sub-acute bacterial endocarditis (blood-poisoning from bacterial colonization of a faulty heart valve) was made, and a trial course of antibiotics was administered without benefit. His general condition steadily deteriorated with persistent low-grade fever. In view of his rapid downhill course a provisional unproved diagnosis of reticulosis (cancer of the lymphatic system) was made, and on 3 November 1977 intravenous ascorbate in a dose regime of 10 g per 24 hours was instituted. Within 36 hours of commencing this form of treatment his clinical status deteriorated alarmingly. From being a very sick man he became nearly moribund, requiring transfer to the intensive care unit. He became extremely confused and vomited constantly, with a sharp fall in his body temperature from the normal value 98.6° to a grossly hypothermic 88.2°F. He also became quite rapidly anemic, requiring blood transfusion. His ascorbate infusion was discontinued and active resuscitation with "space blanket," intravenous hydrocortisone, and general supportive measures succeeded in rescuing him from this perilous situation, so much so that he was allowed home briefly for Christmas. He was readmitted on 27 December, still undiagnosed, with recurrence of fever, progressive enlargement of the liver and spleen, and increasing jaundice, leading to his death in late January 1978. The correct diagnosis was revealed only at autopsy: he had extensive abdominal Hodgkin's disease, the commonest form of malignancy of the lymphatic system.

Case Y (cancer of the testicle)

Mr. Y was a 42-year-old railroad booking clerk, who had been previously investigated for infertility and azoospermia (absence of living sperm in his semen). He reappeared in August 1971 with rapidly developing painless enlargement of the left testicle. Orchidectomy (removal of the diseased testicle) was performed, and, as clinically expected, it proved to be malignant. Surgery was followed by a standard course of radiotherapy to the inguinal and para-aortic lymph nodes, but even before this course of treatment had been completed lung metastases had appeared on his chest x-ray photographs. He was readmitted to the hospital in December 1971, still reasonably fit, but with multiple lung metastases and in particular with a large fleshy metastasis growing from the upper gum. (This was in the days before cis-platinum, which now appears to offer significant help in such difficult situations.) He was commenced on intravenous ascorbate, 8 g per day, with disastrous results. Within 36 hours (at which time his ascorbate infusion was stopped) the metastasis within his mouth disintegrated, with hemorrhage that could barely be controlled. He became extremely confused, with high fever, and soon lapsed into unconsciousness, and in spite of all the usual resuscitative measures died some 15 days later. An autopsy was performed and the appearances were quite remarkable. He had innumerable metastases scattered throughout the brain, the lungs, and the abdomen, but the striking feature was that all these metastases were dead, and could easily be scooped out.

Case Z (cancer of the kidney)

We are unsure whether to conclude this chapter with mention of Mr. Z, or even whether Mr. Z should be included in this sub-category. We have decided to do so to illustrate the problems of clinical appraisal in these terminal cancer situations. Mr. Z was a textile packer who had had his left kidney removed for cancer in 1967 and who developed lung metastases in 1968, but who then enjoyed considerable benefit from hormone therapy and, later, chemotherapy. By early 1972, however, time for Mr. Z was clearly running out, with the presence of innumerable visceral and skeletal metastases. Although the outlook for Mr. Z was clearly hopeless, he was not judged to be at the point of death. In his tattered dressing gown he was busy around our ward helping people he thought less fortunate than himself. On the day before his planned dismissal he was started on oral ascorbate, 10 g per day. Within 36 hours he suffered an epileptiform convulsion with steadily rising fever and signs of intracranial hemorrhage, leading to death in deep coma some three days later. Although in this patient autopsy permission was not obtained, there seems little doubt that the immediate cause of death was hemorrhage from brain metastases, and there is strong circumstantial evidence that the administration of ascorbate was the precipitating factor in this situation.

Tumor hemorrhage and necrosis, although quite disastrous for these three patients, are in fact evidence of the very strongest defensive response, and would have been a very desirable reaction in patients with earlier and smaller lesions. It would seem that as a result of giving ascorbate all of the tumor cells died, and the reason that these patients became so profoundly ill was that their bodies simply could not cope with the sudden task of getting rid of such a large mass of dead tissue. We can only surmise as to why ascorbate had such a pronounced effect on these three patients but is apparently innocuous in all the others. These three patients were all suffering from far advanced disease, with a very considerable total tumor load. Moreover, they were suffering from highly aggressive rapidly-dividing tumors. We visualize a situation of these masses of tumor cells dividing at the very limits of their nutritional resources, relying heavily upon hyaluronidase-assisted diffusion to supply these needs, and the sudden cut-off, induced by ascorbate, was sufficient to bring about abrupt tumor cell death. The possibility of such a reaction is clearly a matter of great importance to any cancer patient contemplating taking vitamin C. First we would like to emphasize the rarity of this type of reaction; we know of its occurrence in only six patients out of over 500. Secondly, it would seem to occur only in patients with far advanced disease, where the tumor is particularly rapidly growing. Finally, as an additional precaution, we now advise patients starting on vitamin C to introduce the regime by a gradual dose schedule. One gram the first day, 2 grams the second day, and so forth until the required dose, usually between 10 and 20 grams per day, is reached. Since the introduction of this precaution no further adverse reactions of this type have been encountered.

Patients with advanced cancer contemplating a vitamin C regime are understandably eager to know which of the six categories of response they might expect. We find that we cannot make reliable predictions, but there is a trend for the more beneficial responses to be seen in the more rapidly growing tumors, such as Hodgkin's disease, reticulum cell sarcoma, and very vascular tumors. The frequency of individual responses is also difficult to define because of the very considerable overlap between the adjacent categories. A cautious estimate would be as follows:

Category 1:	No response	About 20 percent, one in five
Category 2:	Minimal response	About 25 percent, one in four
Category 3:	Tumor retardation	About 25 percent, one in four
Category 4:	Cytostasis (standstill effect)	About 20 percent, one in five
Category 5:	Tumor regression	About 9 percent, just less than one in ten
Category 6:	Tumor death	About 1 percent, one in a hundred

Thus although this treatment might even kill one patient in a hundred (or, to be more strictly correct, accelerate his imminent death), and be of no clear benefit to about one in five such patients, all the remainder would be helped, and in about one in ten the degree of help offered would be very striking indeed. This is a better track record than chemotherapy can boast of in all but a few relatively rare tumors.

Moreover, it is not possible as yet to make a full assessment of the value of ascorbate for patients with advanced cancer. We still do not know the correct dose. Perhaps, as many people have pointed out to us, the results would be even better if larger doses were used.

It must also be remembered that in talking of "results," as explained in the opening paragraphs of this chapter, we can only talk about responses in cancer patients who have reached the end of the road and where all possible treatments have already been tried and exhausted. Logic suggests that the introduction of supplemental ascorbate at much earlier stages in combined treatment regimes would have a much stronger effect. Thus surgery plus ascorbate, radiotherapy plus ascorbate, or hormones plus ascorbate might produce even better results than surgery, radiotherapy, or hormones alone. Chemotherapy plus ascorbate is a more difficult problem. There is no doubt that the ingestion of high doses of ascorbate protects the patient against the unpleasant side effects of anticancer chemotherapy, but there is also the possibility that the ascorbate may be protecting the tumor against the poisoning effect of the chemotherapeutic drug. Research at the Linus Pauling Institute is being carried out in the hope of elucidating this problem. Until we know more we can offer only speculative advice. We suggest that in the few rare forms of cancer that can be cured by aggressive chemotherapy it is probably wise *not* to take ascorbate during each treatment cycle, in order to allow the drug to exert its full action, and then to take ascorbate between courses to restore the depletion caused by the illness and accentuated by the treatment. When chemotherapy is being given for palliation rather than for cure, we believe that patients should also take high doses of ascorbate at the same time. The ascorbate may diminish the cytotoxic effects of the chemotherapy to a certain extent, but this effect should be more than counterbalanced by the beneficial effect exerted by the ascorbate, and at least the patient will find the chemotherapy courses to be much more tolerable. In this way we return to our basic therapeutic objective, to permit the patient to live out his life in comfort and dignity.

21

Some Illustrative Patients from the United States and Canada

Our publications in the medical and scientific literature advancing the view that supplemental ascorbate is of some value to all cancer patients and can be dramatically beneficial to a fortunate few have received some publicity in the lay press. As a result an unknown but probably rather large number of cancer patients throughout the world are now taking ascorbate in regular high dosages. In addition, many advanced cancer patients, or their close relatives, have written or telephoned us seeking help. This correspondence contains a disproportionately high number of doctors deeply concerned about their own illness or a similar illness in some close relative. In our replies we have always stressed that the attending physician, familiar with all the clinical details, is the person best qualified to make treatment decisions, but have added our belief that supplemental ascorbate is compatible with all conventional forms of cancer treatment and should be of some help.

We have received no further communication from many of these patients and we must assume that they derived no appreciable benefit from ascorbate or were dissuaded by their physicians from its use. It is possible that this may be an over-cautious appreciation of the true situation, as the following example illustrates. In July 1976 we received a letter from a nurse in New York very concerned about her father in Portland, Oregon, who was dying from lung cancer with visceral and skeletal metastases. We responded but received no reply. We recently learned from another cancer patient in Portland that this first man is now quite well "as expected," but three postal requests for specific information to the daughter at her last known address remain unanswered.

We must still accept that this Portland man and his untraceable daughter are exceptional, and that the non-responders were not helped. This leaves a scattered and self-selected group of far advanced cancer patients who claim to have derived appreciable benefit. We are well aware that "placebo" and "anticipation" effects could be playing an important part in such reports.

In a relentlessly progressive fatal illness such as cancer, however, where the chance of spontaneous remission has been estimated to be less than 1 in 100,000, it seems clear to us that such a chance is very much improved in the comparatively few cancer patients who have elected to boost their own resistance by ingesting supplemental ascorbate in adequate dosage.

The first patient described in the following paragraphs was reported in the medical literature in the 1950s, long before our own interest in this subject was aroused. The remaining patients presented in this chapter come from our own files, and are given with each patient's permission and after verification by perusal of the patient's medical records. Such anecdotal accounts have no statistical value; nevertheless, they seem to us to have some significance.

Case A′ (chronic myeloid leukemia)

In 1954 Dr. Edward Greer, of Robinson, Illinois, published a report about a remarkable patient who apparently controlled his cancer (chronic myeloid leukemia) over a period of two years by the oral intake of very large amounts of vitamin C. This patient, an elderly executive of an oil company, had a number of concurrent illnesses. He developed chronic heart disease in September 1951 and was described in May 1952 as having alcoholic cirrhosis of the liver and polycythemia (an increased number of circulating red blood cells). In August 1952 the diagnosis of chronic myeloid leukemia was established and verified by an independent hematologist. In September 1952, after extraction of some of his teeth, he was advised to take some vitamin C to promote healing of his gums. He immediately began to take very large amounts, from 24.5 g to 42 g per day (seven 500-mg tablets taken 7 to 12 times a day). He said that he set this regime for himself because he felt so much better when he took these very large doses. The patient repeatedly remarked about his feeling of well-being, and he continued to work as a company executive. On two occasions Dr. Greer insisted that the vitamin C be stopped. Both times when this was done the patient's spleen and liver became enlarged, soft, and tender, his temperature rose to 101°, and he complained of general malaise and fatigue, typical leukemic symptoms. His signs and symptoms rapidly improved when the intake of vitamin C was resumed. He died of acute cardiac decompensation in March 1954, at age 73. His spleen was then firm, and the leukemia, polycythemia, cirrhosis, and myocarditis had shown no progression during the 18 months since he began his intake of large doses of vitamin C. Greer concluded that "the intake of the huge dose of ascorbic acid appeared to be essential for the welfare of the patient."

Case B' (carcinoma of the pancreas)

A 50-year-old housewife in British Columbia, Canada, developed painless jaundice in May 1978. Pre-operative CAT-scans demonstrated a tumor 6 cm in diameter in the head of the pancreas, obstructing the common bile duct. At surgery, the same month, the diagnosis of pancreatic cancer was confirmed and the tumor was judged to be irresectable, the surgeon's notes describing the tumor as being the size of a squash ball. A by-pass procedure was performed to relieve her jaundice. On her own initiative, she commenced taking sodium ascorbate in a dose of 12 to 16 g per day just after her release from hospital, and then increased her intake to 30 g per day in early January 1979. By this time the patient was free of all physical symptoms but had developed reactive depression related to her knowledge of the diagnosis and the predictable prognosis of her inoperable pancreatic cancer. She was referred to a psychiatrist, who encouraged her to continue with her high ascorbate intake. Two repeat CAT-scans were carried out in February 1979 and March 1979, and to everyone's surprise they showed no evidence of any residual pancreatic tumor. The patient continues to take 30 g of sodium ascorbate per day, she remains fit and well, and she is understandably no longer depressed about her illness.

Case C' (brain tumor)

The 55-year-old wife of a California physician gradually became aware of difficulty in coordinating the fine movement of her right hand. Although she taught Japanese brush painting as a hobby, her first awareness of the problem was inexplicable difficulty in writing checks and even signing her own name to these checks in the supermarket. These rather vague symptoms commenced somewhere around July or August 1978, and steadily progressed to partial weakness of the whole right arm, some weakness of the right leg, a partial facial paresis, and increasing difficulty in speaking and in swallowing because of inability to coordinate the movements of her tongue. Within a matter of weeks she was considerably disabled. She consulted a leading neurosurgeon at Stanford Medical Center in September 1978, who, on the basis of her symptoms, her abnormal neurological signs, and the clear evidence of a brain scan, made a firm diagnosis of a 2.5-cm-diameter tumor lying deep in the left cerebral hemisphere. On the clear evidence before him, the neurosurgeon correctly advised immediate operation, but warned her that because of the anatomical location of the tumor she would be left with a permanent degree of hemiparesis (paralysis of the right arm and leg). The prospect terrified her, and she refused to accept this advice. She consulted another experienced neurosurgeon, who independently confirmed the diagnosis of brain tumor and made the same strong recommendation for immediate life-saving surgery. Again she refused, in spite of her husband's worried insistence. At this point she was becoming desperate. On a relative's suggestion, gleaned from a newspaper article, she commenced taking vitamin C in September 1978 at a dose of 10 grams per day. She now freely admits that this was an act of despair and that she did not really expect any benefit to ensue.

By late October 1978 she was aware of some symptomatic improvement, with some return of power and coordination in her right arm and leg, and a repeat brain-scan carried out at that time showed that the tumor had not only diminished somewhat in size but had acquired a somewhat fuzzy outline and a somewhat fragmented appearance. Her symptomatic improvement continued and by late December 1978 no evidence of any tumor could be seen on a repeat brain-scan. The patient remains fit and extremely well, still taking 10 grams of vitamin C per day, and appears to have made a virtually complete recovery from her life-threatening illness. A barely noticeable drooping of one corner of her mouth is the only obvious residual disability. She is regarded by her neurosurgeons at Stanford Medical Center as having enjoyed a complete "spontaneous" regression.

Case D' (breast cancer with multiple skeletal metastases)

An elderly woman, living in a retirement community in Florida with her husband, was totally bedridden and in severe pain in January 1978 because of widespread skeletal and visceral metastases from breast cancer. At this point she commenced taking sodium ascorbate, rapidly building up to an intake of 24 g per day. She experienced appreciable relief from intolerable bone pain and was soon able to enjoy short walks along the beach with her husband. However, this relief proved to be very short-lived. Liver metastases that were known to be present expanded, producing portal-vein obstruction with tense ascites, and after a very rapid downhill course, during which time she was unable to take any supplemental vitamin C, she died from extensive carcinomatosis in late March 1978.

Case E' (metastatic carcinoma of the prostate)

In March 1976 a 69-year-old retired executive living near Carmel, California, was found to have cancer of the prostate. This was treated by local irradiation with good effect and the patient commenced taking ascorbic acid, 1 g per day.

In July 1978, however, he developed severe backache and was found to have quite extensive skeletal metastases. The disease was treated by bilateral orchidectomy (to reduce male hormone production) and palliative radiotherapy to the thoraco-lumbar spine. At this point the patient increased his ascorbate regime to 6 g per day. The total therapeutic response has been excellent and this patient is now clinically, radiologically, and biochemically free of malignant disease. Such an excellent therapeutic response could, of course, be attributed to the orchidectomy alone, but we suspect that the ascorbate has contributed to the happy outcome.

Case F' (leukemia)

A 40-year-old hospital engineer in San Francisco was forced into premature retirement on the grounds of ill health in 1974. His complaints were of steadily increasing lassitude and constant bone pain. Initially he was wrongly diagnosed as suffering from aplastic anemia, and he was treated by steroids and repeated blood transfusions as required. His condition continued to deteriorate and further investigations in 1976 including bone marrow biopsy established the correct diagnosis of chronic lymphocytic leukemia of the so-called "hairy cell" (T-lymphocyte) type. He had extensive bone-marrow infiltration with a number of pathological crush fractures of his vertebrae and was considerably disabled. Treatment by steroids was discontinued on the ground that it could be aggravating his osteoporosis. No chemotherapy or radiotherapy was given. The patient himself started to treat his condition in December 1977 with 35 g of vitamin C per day. He claims to have experienced symptomatic relief within a matter of weeks. In April 1978 a splenectomy was performed on the advice of his attending physician.

The patient continues to ingest 35 g of vitamin C per day and remains in complete clinical and hematological remission without any other treatment. While this particular type of leukemia may often pursue a relatively benign and protracted course, there would seem to be little doubt that, in this patient, the transition from a dying to a recovering situation coincided exactly with his commencement of vitamin C. He describes himself now as "the healthiest sick man around," and his physician's most recent note confirms this with the statement "basically has no disease currently." Apart from symptomatic relief, the most striking change since starting suppplemental ascorbate has been a reduction in his blood-transfusion requirements from 6 to 8 pints every five or six weeks to zero, a clear indication that his bone marrow is recovering. The patient is now leading an active life, enjoying his premature retirement, and currently building his own new home in northern California.

Case G' (mycosis fungoides)

The Chief of Pathology at a large hospital in Florida developed an indolent skin rash in 1976, soon followed by discomfort below the left shoulder and what he describes as "spells of peculiar weakness and nausea." A skin biopsy and peripheral blood films were examined by both conventional and electron microscopy by a number of authorities. Some difference of opinion existed, but the majority view, with which the patient himself, an experienced pathologist, concurred, was that the diagnosis was mycosis fungoides. This is a rare form of malignancy arising in the reticulo-endothelial system and related to Hodgkin's disease, which characteristically starts with skin manifestations and then proceeds to systemic involvement. To quote the patient, "Having long heard about high vitamin C therapy, and knowing the dismal features of mycosis fungoides, I began taking 4 grams a day on June 7, 1978; the skin lesions rapidly improved, and within a few months my painful left arm (where x-rays had shown a periostitis [inflammation of the membrane about a bone] accepted to be a systemic manifestation of mycosis fungoides) had completely recovered." At present he is well, apart from a few small residual skin lesions, is actively at work in charge of a large department of pathology, and is still taking 3 g of vitamin C per day. He himself has no doubt about the correctness of the diagnosis and is certain that his improvement has been the direct result of his taking vitamin C.

Case H' (cancer of the bladder)

A 71-year-old man, living in Wisconsin, was first diagnosed as having bladder cancer in 1968. From 1968 until 1975 he had eleven operations (repeated cystodiathermy, repeated transurethral resection) and a course of megavoltage radiotherapy in an attempt to control his disease. During this time he had almost constant hematuria, and he estimates that he "must have bled gallons." In 1975, as a result of reading a magazine article, he began taking 3 g of sodium ascorbate per day. Quite soon thereafter his hematuria ceased abruptly, and it has never recurred. Repeated cystoscopic examinations have shown him to be free of tumor since he started his ascorbate regime.

Case I' (multiple myeloma)

A man living in Florida had become progressively unwell throughout the whole of 1976 with a puzzling illness of increasing weakness, bone pain, and rectal and nasal bleeding. The correct diagnosis of multiple myeloma was established in February 1977. He had a markedly elevated gamma globulin concentration in his blood, a diagnostic feature of this form of malignancy. As soon as the diagnosis was established he began taking ascorbic acid, rapidly building up to a tolerance level of 40 g per day. Within 5 days his rectal bleeding ceased. While still continuing his ascorbic acid, he commenced a 5-drug chemotherapeutic regime, and after 10 months his blood values had returned to normal and a repeat bone-marrow biopsy showed no evidence of any residual myeloma cells. It is interesting to note that as his condition improved his tolerance level for ascorbate fell from 40 to around 20 g per day, indicating a diminished requirement as his disease was brought under control. At the time this man's illness was diagnosed he was in constant pain and barely able to get out of bed; even before chemotherapy was commenced he was aware of distinct symptomatic improvement, and when last heard from he was busily constructing an extension to his home. The skilled chemotherapy undoubtedly contributed to this man's present well-being, but his early response was so rapid and so good that we have no doubt that his vitamin C also contributed to the outcome.

Case J' (lung cancer)

A 50-year-old patient in Milwaukee was found to have cancer of the right lung in August 1977. He had smoked heavily for thirty-two years. A right middle and lower lobectomy (surgical removal of two-thirds of the lung) was performed the same month. The tumor was found to be an undifferentiated squamous-cell epithelioma, a type usually associated with a relatively poor prognosis. His immediate post-operative recovery was quite satisfactory, but in July 1978 a metastasis was discovered in the left lung. Although metastases rarely occur singly, this lesion was also surgically removed and proved to be a metastasis and not a new primary tumor. Soon after the second operation in August 1978 the patient commenced taking 20 g of sodium ascorbate each day, later reduced to 12 g per day. At the time of writing he is reported to be in excellent health, back at work, and enthusiastic about cycling.

Case K' (Hodgkin's disease)

A 29-year-old housewife in West Virginia became progressively unwell throughout 1977 with weight loss, weakness, nausea, and night sweats. Chest x-rays showed a large centrally-placed mediastinal mass, thought at first to be a thyoma. However, at surgery carried out in March 1978 the mass was found to be extensive involvement of the mediastinal lymph glands by Hodgkin's disease. As many glands as possible were removed and the patient was given post-operative radiotherapy. Chemotherapy was strongly advised but refused by the patient, who instead elected to take 10 g of vitamin C per day. Her progress has been much better than expected, and she is now in apparent good health. It is reported in her local newspaper that "if one is up early enough, one might catch a glimpse of this mother of two young children jogging steadily on her mile-long course near her home."

Case L' (lung cancer)

The president of a southern California company, a life-long non-smoker, had a negative chest x-ray in 1974. In November of 1977, while still feeling perfectly well, he commenced taking 10 g of vitamin C per day as a general health measure. Just a few weeks later he was found on routine examination to have an opacity 2.5 cm in diameter in the right lung, suspicious but not absolutely diagnostic of lung cancer. Surgical exploration was advised but, because of the doubt about the diagnosis and his own sense of well-being, it was refused by the patient, who continued his self-prescribed ascorbate regime. Repeat chest x-rays throughout the following year showed no change, increase or decrease, in the size of the lesion. Eventually he was persuaded that surgery was advisable, and in August 1978 a partial pneumonectomy was performed and the lesion was found to be a primary lung cancer. His postoperative recovery is said to have been much faster than normal, with rapid wound healing, and the patient remains fit and well at the time of writing, and a strong advocate of the value of vitamin C. It appears more than possible that the growth of this man's lung cancer was arrested for over nine months, during which time he maintained a regular high ascorbate intake.

Case M' (carcinoma, primary unknown)

In early 1976 a middle-aged Southern Californian had a semi-emergency palliative operation to remove a mass of undifferentiated carcinomatous tissue which had been pressing on the thoracic spinal cord. Prior to surgery he had been unwell for about a year, culminating in total paralysis of both lower limbs and loss of bladder and bowel control. The source of this metastasis was never established. Surgery was followed by radiotherapy to the affected area, and chemotherapy for eighteen months, but throughout that time he made no progress; he could not walk or even turn himself over in bed. Having read a magazine article on the alleged merits of vitamin C, he on his own initiative began taking 10 g per day, and he reports that "inside three weeks I could get out of bed by myself and then I was going from bed to the wheelchair without assistance". Now, nearly three years later, and still on 10 g of vitamin C per day, he appears to have made an almost complete recovery and is playing a vigorous part in his local community affairs.

Case N' (pheochromocytoma)

In 1968 a ski instructor, then only 22 years of age, was operated on for malignant pheochromocytoma, a somewhat rare slow-growing hormone-producing tumor of the adrenal gland. Initially the operation was regarded as being quite successful, but his symptoms gradually recurred and his condition became untreatable by any conventional means. By late 1977 the tumor had recurred locally to compress the vena cava and he was noted to have widespread intra-abdominal metastases. On his own initiative he began taking ascorbic acid, 30 g per day, in January 1978, gradually building up to 80 g per day by March 1979. To quote his own words: "for several years I had lived in unbearable pain and distress," but within a few months he was quite free of pain and able to return to his former activities. He continues well, running a holiday camp in the Sierra for children in the summer months and instructing in winter sports during the season.

Case O' (malignant pleural effusion, primary unknown)

An 83-year-old woman of Allentown, Pennsylvania, was admitted to her local hospital in February 1977 following a gastro-intestinal hemorrhage. X-rays of the alimentary tract disclosed no abnormality other than a "gastric polyp," apparently benign. As an incidental finding, she was discovered to have a left pleural effusion which required to be aspirated on three occasions in a relatively short time, and the aspirated fluid was found on each occasion to contain clumps of typical adenocarcinoma cells. A most thorough investigation by various specialists failed to discover the primary source for her disseminated malignancy, although suspicion must center on the allegedly benign gastric polyp. No treatment was advised. In early March 1977 she began ascorbic acid at the level of 10 g per day and has continued ever since. She remains fit and well, her pleural effusion has never recurred, and regular chest x-rays and serum biochemistry results are always normal.

Case P' (metastatic carcinoma of both lungs)

The elderly wife of a New England artist had a hysterectomy for endometrial cancer 27 years ago, and enjoyed robust health for many years thereafter, and, to quote, "smoking like a chimneystack!" In May 1977 she was hospitalized because of increasing breathlessness and persistent cough, and was found to have tumors in both lungs. The malignant nature of these tumors was confirmed by biopsy, but their precise nature (primary, or metastatic from some unknown primary or from the long-forgotten endometrial cancer) could not be determined with any confidence. The situation was regarded as hopeless and untreatable. While in hospital she commenced taking 15 g of vitamin C per day and at the time of writing, over two years later, she claims to be in perfect health. Serial chest x-rays are reported to show regression of both lung tumors, but we have not yet had the opportunity to examine the original films.

Case Q' (lymphosarcoma)

In November 1976 the 80-year-old mother-in-law of a New Jersey investment banker had emergency surgery for strangulated femoral hernia. During the course of surgery a suspiciously enlarged lymph gland was discovered in the groin; it was removed and was found to be the site of lymphosarcoma. Further investigations including lymphangiography demonstrated extensive involvement of most pelvic and para-aortic lymph nodes (Stage III lymphosarcomatosis). A palliative course of radiotherapy was given without expectation of cure, and the patient herself commenced taking vitamin C, about 10 g per day. At the time of writing, some two and a half years after she began taking vitamin C, this woman pleasurably surprises her therapists by remaining well without any clinical suspicion of any active disease.

Case R' (cancer of the stomach)

The 67-year-old father of a trained nurse was admitted to a hospital in Long Beach in March 1977 following a major gastro-intestinal hemorrhage. It was soon discovered that this had arisen from a carcinoma of the stomach. A partial gastrectomy was carried out; the tumor had already spread to the regional lymph nodes (which were removed) and to the underlying pancreas (which was not). He entered a trial program to try to determine the value of chemotherapy in gastric cancer, but was allocated to the "no-treatment" control group. At his daughter's instigation, he commenced taking 12 g of sodium ascorbate per day around April 1977. His immediate progress was reasonably satisfactory but by October of that year some deterioration was noted. By that time he had fairly clear clinical (nodular enlargement of the cervical lymph nodes) and biochemical (high alkaline phosphatase level) evidence of malignant dissemination. For this he was hospitalized, and, bereft of his vitamin C, he appeared to deteriorate fairly quickly. Again at his daughter's insistence, he was removed from hospital and commenced again on vitamin C, this time at a daily intake of 20 g, steadily increasing to 28 g. The immediate response is said to have been dramatic, with resolution of the enlarged cervical lymph nodes and a sharp drop in his serum alkaline phosphatase levels to the normal range. For the next 16 months he remained well and symptom-free. He was readmitted to his original hospital in Long Beach in April 1979, following an acute attack of gallstone colic. Appropriate radiology demonstrated a diseased gallbladder containing many stones; surgery was performed, the diseased gallbladder was removed, and the surgeon could see no evidence of any residual intra-abdominal malignancy. The patient made an excellent recovery from this second operation, continues to take 28 g of sodium ascorbate a day, and is reported to be enjoying life to the full.

Case S' (brain tumor)

We have failed to obtain the medical and hospital records of this patient, but have little doubt as to the authenticity of the report. The patient is a little boy, now eight years old, living in New Jersey. His mother wrote to us first in February 1978, saying that she had been giving her young son "large doses" of vitamin C for over a year in an apparently successful attempt to restrain his malignant brain tumor. Prior to starting vitamin C in late 1976, the youngster had undergone three unsuccessful surgical attempts to remove the lesion completely, and had had a course of radiotherapy that "didn't help at all" and a course of chemotherapy that was "very rough on his system." By February 1978, after more than a year on vitamin C, repeat brain scans had shown no increase in the size of the tumor, and he was judged by his doctors to be "now stable" and "neurologically in good shape." A request by the authors for details of his further progress elicited a reply from his mother on 22 May 1979 that the little boy "is still doing very well," some two and a half years after being started on vitamin C. The reason why we cannot obtain verification from perusal of the medical records of this particular patient is both absurd and illuminating: the fact that this little lad is ingesting high doses of vitamin C has been kept secret from his doctors, and his mother earnestly requests that this should remain so. In her letters she expresses the wish to be able to make some useful contribution to cancer research but says that "excessive medical bills" preclude any such donation.

Case T' (mesothelioma)

A retired business executive of Calgary, Alberta, then age 77, came to thoracotomy (an operation involving cutting the wall of the chest) in June 1977 after a vague and somewhat indeterminate period of illness. The surgeon's operation notes describe the excision of a tumor of the diaphragmatic pleura which on immediate frozen-section examination was thought to be "highly malignant undifferentiated carcinoma, primary unknown," and multiple other metastatic lesions scattered elsewhere throughout the pleural covering of the lung, a few of which were biopsied and found to show the same microscopic appearance. A more leisurely and thorough microscopic examination of the resected tumor and the biopsies of the other lesions established the final diagnosis of malignant mesothelioma of the pleura. No further treatment was advised in such a notoriously hopeless situation, other than three injections of 5-fluorouracil at weekly intervals, which evoked considerable systemic upset including a widespread skin reaction.

On his own initiative, this patient began taking supplemental ascorbate on 3 July 1977, starting at 10 g per day and quickly building up to 25 g per day by 17 July, the level he has maintained ever since. When last heard from, in late May 1979, this patient remained fit and well, with repeated chest x-rays, isotope study of the liver, and CAT brain scans showing no trace of any active disease. As a deeply concerned layman, he has written to the Canadian authorities some highly perceptive proposals as to how proper therapeutic trials of cancer should be conducted. A response is still awaited.

Case U' (disseminated breast cancer)

We include the following story to illustrate the dangers of accepting anecdotal evidence at face value. A charming 69-year-old woman living in the timber country near the California-Oregon border had a mastectomy for Stage-II breast cancer in June 1975. Towards the end of 1976 she developed an expanding painful metastasis in the bony pelvis, confirmed by plain radiography and isotope bone scan. She then began high daily intakes of vitamin C, and two years later reported enthusiastically that her pain had been dramatically relieved and that a repeat bone scan had shown the skeletal metastases to be very much reduced in size. We have since acquired her medical records, which confirm all these statements. However, we discovered that she had failed to mention that during the same period the pelvic metastasis had been surgically curetted, that the metastatic breast-cancer cells had been found to have estrogen receptors, that she had been treated with estrogens, and that palliative radiotherapy had been given to the painful area. Her overall beneficial response must certainly be attributed in large part to these conventional measures, but this does not mean that her supplemental ascorbate played no beneficial role. At the time of writing, there has been a very slow progression of her illness in spite of continuing with estrogens and ascorbate and further courses of palliative radiotherapy.

Case V' (disseminated prostatic cancer)

A retired U.S. Navy admiral and decorated veteran of the Battles of Midway and Coral Sea was diagnosed in January 1971 as having prostatic cancer, confirmed by biopsy. Stilbestrol was advised but refused by the patient because of lack of symptoms and its possible feminizing effects. By late 1971 the tumor was judged by his urologist to be progressing and the patient began taking vitamin C, 8 g per day. By March 1972 the primary tumor was judged to be somewhat smaller, and the patient reduced his vitamin C intake to 1 g per day. By mid 1974 the urologist considered that the tumor was again progressing and strongly advised local radiotherapy, but this was refused by the patient, who instead increased his vitamin C intake to 10 g daily together with oral Laetrile. He remained virtually symptom-free until the spring of 1978, when a transurethral resection of the prostatic tumor was required to alleviate bladder-neck obstruction and when a bone scan indicated metastases in the bony pelvis. The patient refused estrogens and increased his vitamin C intake to 12 g per day. Metastatic bone pain continued intermittently over the summer months of 1978, with steady increase in the serum acid phosphatase level, clearly indicating progressive malignant activity. Treatment by estrogens was strongly advised but again refused by the patient, who instead increased his daily vitamin C intake to 20 g. In October 1978 he sought treatment in a private clinic in Jamaica, where in addition to his regular high vitamin C intake he was given high doses of vitamin A and placed on a strict vegetarian diet, apparently with good effect. He suffered a stroke in April 1979, but has recovered nearly completely and is again active and apparently free of symptoms of cancer. The management of this patient, decided by himself, has been quite unorthodox and inadvisable—it is almost certain that he would have derived considerable benefit from estrogens, as originally recommended. However, he, at age 78, does represent an example of prostatic cancer maintained under reasonable control for a period of over eight years without the benefit of hormonal measures, and with the fluctuating activity of his cancer directly related to his level of ascorbate intake.

Case W' (carcinoma of the small intestine)

In February 1975 the 55-year-old wife of a farmer in Ohio had a brain tumor surgically removed. Microscopic examination of the tumor showed it to be a metastatic adenocarcinoma from some unsuspected primary tumor elsewhere. Thorough investigations were carried out at that time but the primary tumor could not be located. The patient began taking a multipurpose vitamin preparation. During 1976 she developed gradually increasing abdominal discomfort, culminating in the need for exploratory surgery, which was carried out in November of that year. A primary adenocarcinoma of the small intestine with metastases to one other part of the small intestine and to the spleen was discovered, and all three intra-abdominal tumors were removed. Immediately following her abdominal surgery she began taking vitamin C, rapidly increasing to a steady intake of 10 to 12 g per day. Two and a half years later, the patient continues in perfect health with no clinical or biochemical evidence of any active malignant disease.

Case X' (lung cancer)

In July 1977 the 72-year-old father of a professor in a technical institute had a pulmonary lobectomy performed for a well-differentiated squamous-cell carcinoma of the right lung. The prognosis was thought to be good, but barely a year later he developed in the opposite lung a tumor that at surgery was found to be irresectable. Following this second operation in August 1978 the patient was given palliative radiotherapy to the left lung tumor and began taking sodium ascorbate, 10 g per day. More recently a regular high intake of vitamin A has been added to this regime. As of June 1979, the patient was clinically well and was described by his son as being "strong and alert." When considered in comparison with the usual rapid downhill course of metastasizing lung cancer, this must be considered as somewhat persuasive evidence that his megavitamin regime is effectively restraining progressive malignant growth.

Case Y' (lung cancer)

A man of 75 living in Oregon was found in January 1978 to have an inoperable carcinoma of the lung involving mediastinal lymph glands and with possible metastasis to the left kidney. Some palliative chemotherapy was given soon after the diagnosis was reached, but it had to be discontinued because of adverse side-effects. He began taking 10 g of ascorbic acid per day in February 1978. Chest x-rays taken in June 1978 showed no appreciable increase or decrease in the size of the tumor, but the patient felt fit enough to embark on a family vacation to Hawaii. By July 1978 repeat chest x-ray examination is reported to show appreciable reduction in the size of the primary lung tumor. The patient has since continued on a high daily ascorbate regime, and at the time of writing, eighteen months after starting ascorbate, he is reported to be in "average" health for a septuagenarian busily tending a 2¼-acre productive garden. It is perhaps worth noting that this patient attributes his continuing good health in part to vitamin C and in part to his active participation in a mutual self-help cancer counseling regime.

Case Z' (disseminated ovarian cancer)

In April 1969 the 47-year-old wife of a biochemist had a hysterectomy and bilateral salpingo-oophorectomy for bilateral ovarian cancer, followed by a standard course of post-operative irradiation. In January 1970 emergency surgery had to be performed for the relief of post-operative adhesions causing intestinal obstruction; no obvious tumor was present at this second operation. Her recovery from this apparently simple mechanical problem was, however, less than satisfactory; her condition steadily deteriorated and further surgery was required in October 1970 for the removal of a mass of metastatic ovarian carcinoma obstructing the colon. Continued symptoms required yet another surgical intervention in late December 1970, when a palliative colostomy was performed to relieve persistent malignant large bowel obstruction. During the course of this operation it was noted that innumerable peritoneal metastases were present. Based on such a finding, a prognosis of six months or less to live was understandably given.

In January 1971, after dismissal from hospital, a palliative course of chemotherapy using Leukeran (chlorambucil) was given and continued for 20 months. At the same time the patient began the regular intake of vitamin C, varying from 3 to 12 g per day adjusted according to bowel tolerance.

In October 1973 further surgery was required for the repair of an incisional hernia and at that time, after 20 months of Leukeran and high Vitamin C ingestion, no evidence of any residual intra-abdominal cancer was found. The chemotherapy was terminated and the patient has continued to ingest the same large amounts of ascorbate through the time of writing, almost six years later. At the present time she is reported to be perfectly fit and well with no suspicion of any active malignant disease. Even the most enthusiastic oncologist would hardly expect a "five-year-cure" in disseminated ovarian cancer from such a relatively low-potency chemotherapeutic agent as Leukeran; we must therefore conclude that her consistent high intake of vitamin C, with undoubted help from her original surgery, her initial post-operative radiotherapy, and her chemotherapy, has contributed to the present happy outcome.

CONCLUSION

This group of patients has been selected from our files to show that supplemental ascorbate appears to have some restraining influence upon a wide variety of malignant tumors. In the present state of our knowledge it is our opinion that supplemental ascorbate is of some value in all forms of cancer and can prove to be of quite dramatic benefit to a fortunate few, as described in this chapter and in the preceding chapter.

The anecdotal evidence given in these two chapters supports our view that supplemental ascorbate should be considered not as an alternative form of cancer treatment but rather as an important supportive measure, with the potential to enhance all well-established cancer therapeutic regimes. Our views about the value of supplemental ascorbate in total cancer management are discussed in the following two chapters.

22

The Prevention of Cancer

The total eradication of cancer from the human race would be the highest goal that world science and medicine could achieve. The benefits to mankind in diminished suffering and healthy productive longevity would be tremendous. The economic benefits would also be staggering in scale. It is a fact that the treatment of a cancer illness in the United States may cost as much as $50,000, and it is well known that the treatment of cancer is the main burden on hospital facilities and health-care personnel in every advanced country in the world. And the cost of cancer research is also reaching astronomic proportions with, to date, little return to show for the huge expenditures. Thus, apart from the degree of suffering and personal misery involved, cancer not only has the real potential to impoverish the family of the unfortunate victim but also devours a significant proportion of national economic resources.

As was mentioned in an earlier chapter, cholera was banished from the city of London by John Snow many years ago not by the discovery of some powerful new treatment, but by discovering and removing the cause—in that case a contaminated water supply. Over the years many other major illnesses have been brought under control and sometimes virtually eliminated by strong preventive measures. In the last few decades three great scourges of mankind, smallpox, poliomyelitis, and tuberculosis, have practically disappeared, through the use of protective vaccinations and the isolation and active treatment of the diminishing number of victims to remove the "cause."

We are entitled to ask whether any such program could be devised to prevent cancer. There is little evidence that cancer is significantly infectious, so that there is no clear need to isolate the victims. The evidence that some human cancers may be caused by a virus remains somewhat tenuous, and the chance of developing a vaccine that would give universal protection against all cancers (like the Salk and Sabin vaccines for poliomyelitis) appears remote. If, however, it did come to pass that such a vaccine were to be developed and brought into practical use, the benefits to mankind would be enormous. Therefore, although the chances of success seem slim, this type of research should be actively pursued and should continue to receive adequate funding.

On a more practical level, while it may not be possible totally to eradicate cancer from the human race, enough information is already known to permit the introduction of important preventive measures that would very significantly reduce its incidence. The practical prevention of cancer requires a two-pronged approach, namely, the reduction of carcinogens in the human environment and the adoption of measures to render our human population more resistant to cancer.

The importance of environmental (including nutritional) factors in causing cancer has been discussed recently by Sir Richard Doll (1977), who summarized the evidence in the following words:

> That environmental factors contribute to the production of the majority of cases with which we have to contend is now obvious, and there is no need to review the evidence in detail. It rests on the great variation in the incidence of most cancers, both from place to place and almost certainly also from time to time; on the experience of migrants, among whom the risk of cancer changes to that of their adopted country in the course of one or two generations; on the recognition every year or so of a new occupational or iatrogenic hazard; and on the discovery that particular types of cancer can be related to specific types of behavior or correlated quantitatively with exposure to a known laboratory carcinogen.

As we have mentioned in Chapter 2, man is under a constant bombardment from a hail of potentially lethal carcinogens. These are a whole variety of physical and chemical agents that share one common property—the ability to interact with and to damage the genetic material of living cells. The usual result of such damage is the inconsequential death of some insignificant cell out of the ten trillion that compose the human body. However, by a million-to-one chance, such damage may rearrange the genetic material in such a way that the offspring of the transformed cell can survive and also acquire malignant characteristics. Therefore the chances of cancer developing increase according to the intensity of the carcinogenic bombardment and the duration of exposure. Today's cancer pandemic arises from a combination of both these factors. Because of lack of knowledge in the past and sometimes because of almost criminal carelessness, there has been a steady increase in the carcinogenic pollution of man's environment, and with the rapid expansion of the chemical industry and other factors this increase has been particularly marked over the last 50 years, and continues to rise. During the same period of time, because of the dramatic advances in almost every other field of medicine, man's expectation of life and therefore duration of exposure to carcinogenic assault has also increased.

The action of carcinogens has tended to focus on the obvious cause-and-effect examples in which cancer develops in an organ or tissue directly exposed to the carcinogenic agent. Such examples are the carcinogenic effect of ultraviolet light on unpigmented skin, of tobacco smoke on the lung mucosa, of nitrosamines on the stomach lining, and of carcinogenic urinary metabolites on the bladder wall. Apart from these well-proven examples of direct or "contact" carcinogenesis, there is an increasingly strong suspicion that exposure to carcinogens can exert a generalized effect. Although absolute proof is lacking, the strong suspicion exists that a person constantly exposed to a carcinogenically polluted environment (such as the food, the water, and even the air in some of our large industrial cities) has an increased general susceptibility to almost every form of cancer. Moreover, many chemicals have only a weak carcinogenic power, but are now present in our environment in such large quantities as probably to make their total cancer-producing effect greater than that of the strong carcinogens.

It is likely that a normal cell or group of cells becomes malignant after several (perhaps five or six) changes in its genetic material. Each change probably involves the action of a single carcinogenic agent—a single molecule or a single photon (a quantum unit of radiation). Studies with animals of the carcinogenicity of chemicals and of radiation are carried out with moderately large doses of the carcinogenic agent. It is found, when the results are analyzed with care, that the carcinogenic effect is proportional to the dose. It is not possible, however, to get significant results for very low doses, because the number of animals required would be enormous. It has been pointed out by Weinhouse, the editor of the leading cancer journal *Cancer Research,* as well as by other authorities that it is difficult to assess the amount of damage done to human beings by the multitude of weak carcinogens, such as various food additives. Usually only a few hundred mice or other animals can be used in a test. In order to get an observable effect (the induction of cancer in some of the animals) rather large doses of a suspected weak carcinogen have to be used. For example, an additive might be present in the food of the average American in the amount of 10 parts per million (10 mg in one kilogram of food). The same amount in the food of 1000 test animals (mice or rats) might cause none of the animals to develop cancer, but when 1 percent of the substance is added to the food it may cause 50 cases of cancer. Although there are many uncertainties, the assumptions are usually made that the carcinogenic effect is proportional to the dose and that a chemical that causes a certain number of cancers in mice or other test animals during their life spans will cause a similar number of cancers in man during his life span. For example, if the weak carcinogen causes 50 cases of cancer in 1000 test animals when 1 percent is added to the food, we expect that an amount one thousand times smaller, 10 parts per million, would cause 50 deaths in 1,000,000 animals, and might well cause 10,000 deaths in the U.S. population. During the 1960s extensive use was made of sodium cyclamate and calcium cyclamate as synthetic sweeteners, replacing sucrose. When it was discovered that the cyclamates cause experimental animals to develop cancer of the bladder this sweetener was banned. Saccharin is now the only synthetic sweetener approved for use in the United States. It, too, has been found to be carcinogenic in animals, and it also may be banned, except for use as a prescription drug. Many other food additives have been found to be carcinogenic and have been banned.

With many thousands of substances to be tested, the determination of their degrees of carcinogenicity presents a tremendous problem. The job has been made simpler by verification of a significant degree of parallelism between carcinogenicity and mutagenicity and the development by Bruce Ames of the University of California in Berkeley of a rather simple and reliable test for mutagenicity (for a review see McCann and Ames, 1977).

The number of cases of cancer caused by a single weakly carcinogenic food additive or other environmental chemical may be small, perhaps a few hundred cases per year; but the combined effect of all of them probably is to cause several tens of thousands of unnecessary deaths among the people of the United States each year. It is well worthwhile to support the efforts of the Food and Drug Administration to identify the carcinogenic substances and to ban them.

There are also actions that the individual human being can take to decrease his own risk of developing cancer. One very important action is for smokers to stop smoking. Every smoker should read about the misery caused by lung cancer, emphysema, and cancer of the lip, tongue, mouth, and larynx, and ask himself if it is necessary that he doom himself to experience this misery.

Also, nonsmokers are damaged when exposed to cigarette, pipe, and tobacco smoke. Recent studies have shown that the nonsmoking wives of smokers have a significantly smaller life expectancy than the nonsmoking wives of nonsmokers. It is beneficial to your health to avoid the company of smokers.

You can achieve a large amount of protection against carcinogenic agents by increasing your intake of vitamin C. This effect of vitamin C is probably in part the result of its general detoxifying action, by which it destroys the carcinogens (Chapter 16) and in part the result of its stimulating the body's natural protective mechanisms (Chapter 15).

Many epidemiological studies have shown the value of foods rich in vitamin C in decreasing the incidence of cancer. (References to the investigations are given by Cameron and Pauling, 1979.) An example is the extensive study by Bjelke (1973, 1974) of 4,888 Norwegian-born men in the United States, 17,818 other men in the United States, and 8,054 men in Norway. Bjelke used questionnaires and interviews to get information about the diet and other factors, and followed the incidence of and mortality from cancer. He found that the most important effect on gastrointestinal cancer was the vitamin C content of the diet: a high total-vegetable intake and a high intake of vitamin C significantly reduced the incidence of gastrointestinal cancer.

An indication of the amount of protection provided by a diet with an increased content is given by the observations of Chope and Breslow (1955) on 577 older people (50 years old or older in 1948) in San Mateo, California, who were studied by questionnaires or interviews and then were checked for seven years for subsequent mortality. Of the many factors correlated with their age-corrected total death rates, mainly from heart disease and cancer, the most important was found to be their intake of vitamin C. Those with a higher intake of vitamin C were found to have a total death rate only 40 percent of that for those with the lower intake (less than 50 mg per day). This decrease in the death rate corresponds to an increase by eleven years in the length of life. Similar but smaller beneficial correlations were found also for two of the B vitamins, pyridoxine (B6) and niacin.

An interesting study, as yet unpublished, of a self-selected cohort of persons interested in health has been made by our colleague Dr. James E. Enstrom, who has given us permission to quote the results. He made a prospective epidemiologic study of 215 male and 150 female California residents who had answered a 1974 questionnaire in *Prevention* magazine and were at least 65 years old at that time. Based on questionnaire information obtained in 1974 and 1977, these people appear to have a healthy lifestyle, including the general avoidance of tobacco, alcohol, sugar, and obesity. Their diet seems to be fairly similar to the average American diet, except that it involves extensive use of dietary supplements, including the average daily intake of about 1,700 mg of vitamin C, 700 I.U. of vitamin E, and 18,000 I.U. of vitamin A, as well as other vitamins and minerals. Their educational and occupational levels are somewhat above average. After 4 years of follow-up of the mortality records, their standardized mortality rate compared with the general California population is 61 percent for the entire cohort and 47 percent for the 293 non-smokers in the group. This mortality rate is among the lowest ever observed in a self-selected elderly population. We believe that it indicates that dietary supplements have a significant influence on health.

In his recent analysis of the origins of human cancer of which we quoted a paragraph at the beginning of this chapter Sir Richard Doll concluded with the words

> In this introduction I have tried to review the main clues to the origin of cancer that have been provided by epidemiologic studies and the way they may interact with laboratory investigations. I have laid particular stress on diet because I suspect that in the next few years the main advances in our knowledge of how to control cancer will come from studying this aspect of our environment.

We agree with this conclusion, and, moreover, we believe that a properly large intake of vitamin C may well be found to be the most important of all dietary factors in the prevention of cancer.

We believe that the officially recommended dietary intake of about 45 mg of vitamin C per day is so much less than the optimum as to constitute in itself a significant cause of cancer. It is our opinion that to keep the age-specific incidence of cancer and of other diseases low it is necessary that the daily intake be at least 250 mg, and for most people a daily intake between 1 g and 10 g per day may lead to the best of health. In addition we recommend a good intake of vitamin A, vitamin E, the B vitamins, and minerals. The daily diet should include good amounts of green, yellow, and red vegetables. The intake of sugar should be kept low. The regime should include eating breakfast every day, not eating between meals, and not overeating. An effort should be made to avoid foods and soft drinks containing possibly carcinogenic dyes and other additives. Some regular daily exercise is helpful, as is 7 or 8 hours of sleep each night. The intake of alcoholic drinks should be kept moderate, and smoking should be absolutely banned.

Adherence to these principles not only increases the chance of living to a ripe old age, but also lengthens the period of well-being, of good health and freedom from cancer and other diseases. You yourself can, by your own decisions, achieve for yourself a happier as well as a longer life than has been the common lot of man and woman in the past.

23

Summary and Conclusions: The Role of Vitamin C in the Treatment of Cancer

The correct treatment of cancer is a matter for almost endless debate, simply because no one knows how to treat cancer correctly. We deplore that increasingly common creature "The Triumphalistic Oncologist," so eloquently caricaturized in the editorial with this title in the journal *Surgery, Gynecology, and Obstetrics* (*146:* 617–618, 1978); his attitude of mind seems to be that in order to introduce any advance in treatment it is first necessary to decry and repudiate any advance that has gone before.

Such a self-serving approach is clearly ludicrous; it deliberately ignores the established fact that conventional treatments, based on either scientific fact or empirical discoveries, can *cure* at least one third of all cancer patients, essentially controlling their disease to such an extent as to given them normal life expectancy. The real objective is to see whether this successful fraction can be even marginally increased by the correct use of all therapeutic resources. Every day, 1100 citizens of the United States die of cancer. If it were possible to decrease this number by even one-tenth, this would mean the saving of 110 lives a day, 770 a week, 3300 a month, and 40,000 in the course of a year.

We firmly believe that supplemental ascorbate used correctly alongside conventional methods of treating cancer has very much greater potential than that.

CHAPTER 23

It seems abundantly clear that ascorbic acid is directly involved in many of the natural mechanisms that protect an individual against cancer. Cancer itself, as we have seen, depletes the body's stores of ascorbate and is almost always associated with some measurable impairment of its immune mechanisms. Therefore, as a matter of principle, no matter what form of established cancer treatment is employed, active steps should be taken to ensure that the patient's ascorbate reserves are constantly kept high in order to allow his protective immune system to function always at maximum efficiency.

The value of surgery in the treatment of cancer is beyond dispute. If the tumor is still localized to an organ or tissue that can be safely excised without undue risk to the patient, such a step is undoubtedly the treatment of choice. "Cut it out and throw it away" may seem to be a most primitive and unsophisticated approach, but it is still far and away the most effective treatment we have.

VITAMIN C AND SURGERY

During the course of cancer surgery clumps of malignant cells can very frequently be found in the peripheral blood; for instance, in a sample drawn from an arm vein during the course of an abdominal operation. These clumps of malignant cells have been literally squeezed out of the tumor by the surgeon's handling. Each such clump has the potential to form a metastasis, but very few of them do so, most of them being overcome by the host's defensive mechanisms. It has long been recognized that surgical resections and even surgical biopsies pose some risk of disseminating metastases. It is our belief, based on the arguments presented in this book, that it is essential to cover this highly critical period of possible tumor dissemination by the provision of adequate ascorbate to ensure that the immune mechanisms are in peak condition.

Unless positive steps are taken to ensure this, the exact reverse holds true.

Any physical or psychic trauma depletes the ascorbate reserves, and the degree of depletion is directly proportional to the extent of the trauma. Any surgical operation is traumatic, and by its very nature surgery for cancer tends to be major, involving much tissue trauma and an appreciable reduction in the body's stores of available ascorbate. The situation is further complicated by the fact that during the course of most major operations for cancer supportive blood transfusion is required, and stored blood contains no ascorbate. To make matters even worse, many major procedures for cancer of the gastrointestinal tract are preceded by a period of enforced starvation to clear the intestine of fecal content, as well as a similar period post-operatively to reduce the risks of peritonitis from a leaking anastomosis. Thus a patient starting with cancer, bereft of his usual dietary sources of vitamin C for several days, subjected to the trauma of major cancer surgery, and perhaps with half of his circulating blood-volume replaced by ascorbate-free stored blood, will have an appreciable reduction in his ascorbate reserves and particularly in the ascorbate content of his circulating lymphocytes at the very time of high risk when a surplus is required.

Ascorbate has other values for the cancer patient undergoing surgery. As has been mentioned in earlier chapters, it has long been known that adequate amounts of ascorbate are essential for the proper healing of wounds and to enhance the defensive mechanisms against bacterial infection. Many major cancer operations on patients depleted of ascorbate by all the mechanisms noted above can be technically perfect but still the patient may be plagued by serious and sometimes fatal post-operative complications. Such complications include partial or complete wound rupture or rupture of some internal anastomosis with peritonitis, wound infections, pneumonia, and cystitis. It is our belief that many of these all too common complications could be prevented if steps were taken to ensure that all such patients were maintained in positive ascorbate balance throughout the whole peri-operative period. The ways of doing this are given in Appendix IV.

VITAMIN C AND RADIOTHERAPY

As discussed in an earlier chapter, the value of radiotherapy in many forms of cancer is beyond dispute, whether it be used alone or as a complement to surgery. Irradiation, however, also produces an appreciable reduction in ascorbate reserves, and general principles suggest that such a deficit should be rectified or even prevented by increasing the ascorbate intake throughout the whole period of treatment.

There is some evidence, dating back to the 1940s, to the effect that patients on relatively high vitamin C intake suffer fewer unpleasant side-effects during treatment by radiotherapy, and also that high vitamin C intake increases the therapeutic value of the high-energy radiation. An especially significant study is that of Cheraskin and his associates (Chapter 19), who found a significantly better response in 27 patients with squamous-cell carcinoma of the uterine cervix who were given 750 mg of ascorbic acid per day during radiation treatment than in 27 similar patients who received the radiation treatment without the ascorbic acid.

Radiotherapy destroys a fairly large volume of tissue and its effects can be likened to those of a deep burn. The cells and other exposed tissue structures disintegrate and die, forming toxic breakdown products that have to be carried off by the bloodstream and excreted in the urine. It is believed that the unpleasant systemic side-effects of radiotherapy (nausea, lassitude) are caused by this sudden metabolic overload of toxic by-products. Ascorbic acid is essential for the proper functioning of a group of liver enzymes concerned with the detoxification and disposal of noxious substances, and it is therefore quite possible that a high intake of ascorbate reduces the unpleasant side-effects of irradiation.

In its anticancer role, high-energy radiation kills cells during their most vulnerable phase of cell division. It is believed that the cell-killing mechanism is the chemical attack on cellular DNA by free radicals produced by the ionizing effect of radiation on the tissues. Free radicals are highly reactive unstable compounds, containing an odd number of electrons, and because of their reactivity they can exist only briefly in the tissues. It is known that ascorbate reacts in the tissues with molecular oxygen to form free radicals, and it is accordingly possible that a high tissue level of ascorbate would potentiate the cytotoxic effect of irradiation. It is certainly known that the therapeutic effects of irradiation can be intensified by increasing the degree of oxygen saturation in the tissues, and this effect is utilized to good effect in the radiation treatment of patients in hyperbaric oxygen chambers.

Apart from its cytotoxic action, radiotherapy exerts a therapeutic effect against cancer in another way. The ground substance of the whole area irradiated is replaced by a much more dense collagenized area of scar tissue. This produces a much more hostile and impermeable environment for any stray cancer cells that have survived the killing effect of the radiation. Ascorbate is, of course, essential for the production of collagen, and an adequate ascorbate supply would ensure that this scirrhous response to radiation would reach its maximum intensity. We conclude that there are no contraindications to taking high levels of vitamin C during radiotherapy; and that, on the contrary, there are a number of strong arguments that such a combination would be beneficial.

VITAMIN C AND HORMONAL TREATMENT

There are no known contraindications to the use of ascorbate alongside any hormonal treatment used in the control of cancer, and we have many patients under treatment by such combinations as DES plus ascorbate, Tamoxifen plus ascorbate, and steroids plus ascorbate. It is our observation that these patients benefit significantly from the inclusion of vitamin C in their treatment.

VITAMIN C AND IMMUNOTHERAPY

We have stated earlier (Chapters 9 and 15) our view that the effectiveness of immunotherapy would be substantially advanced if the patients were at the same time ingesting high levels of ascorbate. The therapeutic use of vitamin C in fact might be considered to be mainly an example of immunotherapy, although this vitamin also exercises many functions in addition to that of potentiating the immune mechanisms. We see no reason for not using vitamin C together with immunotherapy.

VITAMIN C AND CHEMOTHERAPY

The question of the use of ascorbate with chemotherapy is difficult to answer, and much more research is required in this field. In the first place, it seems clear from our own observations and from the many personal reports we have received from others that patients taking high doses of vitamin C are spared many of the unpleasant side-effects of cancer chemotherapy regimes. In a few patients this has allowed doses of chemotherapeutic drugs much larger than usual to be used to good effect. The worry is that ascorbic acid, acting as a general detoxifying agent, may be protecting not only the patient but also his tumor against the poisoning effect of these drugs. This may be a somewhat over-cautious concern. It has recently been reported in tissue-culture studies that sodium ascorbate actually potentiates the cell-killing effect of a number of cytotoxic drugs in common use, with the exception of methotrexate, whose effects were reduced.

By its very nature, cancer chemotherapy depresses the whole immune system, and, as well as reducing the number of circulating lymphocytes, it also produces a sharp fall in the ascorbate content of each individual lymphocyte, hence reducing its protective capacity. There is therefore a strong argument that patients on cancer chemotherapy regimes should protect their immune status by taking large amounts of vitamin C. Until the worry that vitamin C might be reducing the effectiveness of the cancer chemotherapeutic drugs is resolved, we suggest the following course of action for patients with cancers of the sort that respond reasonably well to chemotherapy. Cancer chemotherapy is often given in courses lasting 24 to 48 hours at intervals of three to four weeks. The drugs used in cancer chemotherapy act fairly rapidly and are quickly eliminated from the body. Therefore we suggest that during the 24 to 48 hours of intensive treatment vitamin C be withheld, but recommenced in high dosage during the whole treatment-free interval to restore the ascorbate status and to salvage the damage to the immune system. We must

stress that the interaction between ascorbate and these drugs is really unknown, and research may well show that they act synergistically—that is,
cancer chemotherapy may have increased effectiveness in patients concurrent-
ly taking high levels of vitamin C.

One circumstance seems abundantly clear. If a cancer patient has been
treated by chemotherapy to the point of bone-marrow failure and complete
collapse of his immune system, giving ascorbate at that point is hardly likely
to do much good, because a principal mode of action of ascorbate is by
increasing the power of the immune system, and a badly damaged immune
system may not be able to respond. This conclusion, that vitamin C is far less
effective in patients with advanced cancer whose immune systems have been
badly damaged by extensive courses of chemotherapy, seems to be supported
by the results of the Mayo Clinic trial, as discussed in Chapter 19.

An important question that needs to be answered is whether an adult patient
with a solid malignant tumor that has not been controlled by other treatments
should, as the last resort, receive chemotherapy or ascorbate. A valuable
summary of current opinion of the use of chemotherapy in the treatment of
gastrointestinal cancer has been published in *The New England Journal of
Medicine* (9 November 1978) by Moertel. He pointed out that two decades
ago the fluorinated pyrimidines 5-fluorouracil (5-FU) and 5-fluoro-2'-
deoxyuridine were found to be capable of producing a transient decrease of
tumor size in patients with metastatic cancer of intestinal origin. An intravenous treatment in amount that produces toxic reactions is the most effective,
but the effect is not great:

> Even when administered in most ideal regimens, the fluorinated pyrimidines, in a
> large experience, will produce objective response in only about 15 to 20 percent
> of treated patients. In this context, objective response is usually defined as a
> reduction of more than 50 percent in the product of longest perpendicular dia-
> meters of a measurable tumor mass. These responses are usually only partial and
> very transient, persisting for a median time of only about five months. This minor
> gain for a small minority of patients is probably more than counterbalanced by the
> deleterious influence of toxicity for other patients and by the cost and inconveni-
> ence experienced by all patients. There is no solid evidence that treatment with
> fluorinated pyrimidines contributes to the over-all survival of patients with
> gastrointestinal cancer regardless of the stage of the disease at which they are
> applied.

Moertel also discusses the clinical trials of 5-FU and other chemotherapeutic agents singly and in various combinations in relation to colorectal cancer,
gastric carcinoma, squamous-cell carcinoma of the esophagus, and others,
with essentially the same conclusion except that adriamycin seems to have

significant value for the treatment of primary liver cancer. He then states that "In 1978 it must be concluded that there is no chemotherapy approach to gastrointestinal carcinoma valuable enough to justify application as standard clinical treatment."

We would interpret this conclusion as sound reason for not subjecting these patients to the misery, trouble, and expense of chemotherapy, but in fact Moertel continues as follows:

> By no means, however, should this conclusion imply that these efforts should be abandoned. Patients with advanced gastrointestinal cancer and their families have a compelling need for a basis of hope. If such hope is not offered, they will quickly seek it from the hands of quacks and charlatans. Enough progress has been made in chemotherapy of gastrointestinal cancer so that realistic hope can be generated by entry of those patients into well designed clinical research studies. . . . If we can channel our efforts and resources into constructive research programs of sound scientific design, we shall offer the most hopeful treatment for the patient with gastrointestinal cancer today and lay a sound foundation for chemotherapy approaches of substantive value for the patient of tomorrow.

We do not agree with this conclusion. For more than a decade it has been the rather general practice in Vale of Leven Hospital and most other hospitals in Britain not to subject patients with advanced gastrointestinal cancer and similar cancers for which experience has shown chemotherapy to have little value to the misery of this treatment; instead, these "hopeless" patients were given only palliative treatment, including morphine and heroin as needed to control pain. Now, however, there is a real reason for these patients and their families to have hope. These "untreatable" patients can be given supplemental ascorbate as their only form of treatment and derive some benefit, and just occasionally the degree of benefit obtained might be quite remarkable, as several of the patients described in the preceding chapters illustrate. The average increase in survival time of patients with advanced gastrointestinal cancer treated with 10 g of ascorbate per day is greater than that reported by Moertel for those treated with chemotherapy, and the ascorbate-treated patients have the advantages of feeling well under the treatment and of not having the financial burden of chemotherapy. Moreover, little effort has been made as yet to determine the most effective dosages of vitamin C and the possible supplementary value of vitamin A, the B vitamins, minerals, and a diet high in fruits, vegetables, and their juices. This nutritional treatment of cancer, with emphasis on vitamin C, is probably far more effective at earlier stages of cancer than in the terminal stage, and if it is instituted at the first sign of cancer it may well decrease the cancer mortality by much more than our earlier estimate of 10 percent.

CONCLUSION

With the possible exception of during intense chemotherapy, we strongly advocate the use of supplemental ascorbate in the management of all cancer patients from as early in the illness as possible. We believe that this simple measure would improve the overall results of cancer treatment quite dramatically, not only by making the patients more resistant to their illness but also by protecting them against some of the serious and occasionally fatal complications of the cancer treatment itself. We are quite convinced that in the not too distant future supplemental ascorbate will have an established place in all cancer-treatment regimes.

Appendix I

Estimated Cancer Deaths in the United States for 1980*

Site	Total	Male	Female
All sites	407,320	219,290	188,030
Buccal cavity and pharynx	9,160	6,360	2,800
Lip	185	160	25
Tongue	2,075	1,450	625
Mouth	2,700	1,750	950
Pharynx	4,200	3,000	1,200
Digestive organs	107,800	56,880	50,920
Esophagus	7,250	5,300	1,950
Stomach	14,950	8,800	6,150
Small intestine	720	360	360
Colon	43,100	20,200	22,900
Rectum	10,150	5,550	4,600
Liver and biliary passages	9,800	4,700	5,100
Pancreas	20,550	11,200	9,350
Other digestive	1,280	770	510
Respiratory system	106,100	76,300	29,800
Larynx	3,700	2,900	800
Lung	101,000	72,500	28,500
Other respiratory	1,400	900	500
Bone, tissue, and skin	9,430	5,230	4,200
Bone	1,850	1,030	820
Connective tissue	1,640	820	820
Skin	5,940	3,380	2,560
Breast	35,000	300	34,700

(continued on page 198)

Site	Total	Male	Female
Genital organs	45,280	22,150	23,130
Uterine cervix, invasive	7,600	—	7,600
Uterine corpus, endometrium	3,380	—	3,380
Ovary	11,100	—	11,100
Prostate	21,100	21,100	—
Other genital, male	1,050	1,050	—
Other genital, female	1,050	—	1,050
Urinary organs	17,750	11,800	5,950
Bladder	10,180	7,100	3,080
Kidney and other urinary	7,570	4,700	2,870
Eye	400	200	200
Brain and central nervous system	9,500	5,000	4,500
Endocrine glands	1,600	570	1,030
Thyroid	1,130	310	820
Other endocrine	470	260	210
Leukemia	15,500	8,700	6,800
Lymphomas including multiple myeloma	22,000	11,800	10,200
Lymphosarcoma and reticulo-sarcoma	7,000	3,700	3,300
Hodgkin's disease	2,630	1,500	1,130
Multiple myeloma	6,000	3,000	3,000
Other lymphomas	6,370	3,600	2,770
All other and unspecified sites	27,800	14,000	13,800

*This table has been prepared by extrapolation from the 1978 table of E. Silverberg, *CA — A Cancer Journal for Clinicians, 28,* 17–30, 1978, and other sources.

Appendix II

Foods and Nutrition

During the middle part of the 19th century chemists showed that the principal constituents of foods are *carbohydrates, fats,* and *proteins*. It was recognized that food proteins, when they are digested, provide amino acids, which are the building blocks for the proteins of the human body, including the structural proteins of muscle, tendons, bone, blood vessels, and skin, and the globular proteins, such as hemoglobin and various enzymes. The carbohydrates and fats, as well as the proteins, provide energy, through their combustion in the cells of the body. Then in the period around 1880 it was shown that *minerals* (compounds of metals) are also required for life. Sodium, potassium, magnesium, and calcium are present as ions in the blood and intercellular fluids. Iron is present in the hemoglobin of the blood and in other proteins. In addition, copper, zinc, manganese, chromium, vanadium, silicon, selenium, molybdenum, and tin are all required in small amounts for life. *Nonmetallic elements* are also needed. Chlorine is present as chloride ion in the blood and intercellular fluids. Phosphorus is found as phosphate ion in the blood, as compounds of phosphoric acid in the blood and tissues, and as calcium hydroxyphosphate in the bones and teeth. Sulfur is an important part of many proteins.

Biochemists, physiologists, biostatisticians, and medical investigators have worked hard to determine what intakes of the various constituents of foods are needed for life and good health. The problem is a difficult one, because people are not all the same in their genetic nature and in their requirements. In the United States official recommendations about the intakes (recommended dietary allowances, RDAs) are made by the Food and Nutrition Board of the National Academy of Sciences and National Research Council. (Similar recommendations, usually somewhat larger, have also been made by the Food and Drug Administration of the Department of Health, Education, and Welfare.) Values of the RDAs for many nutrients are shown in Figure II-1.

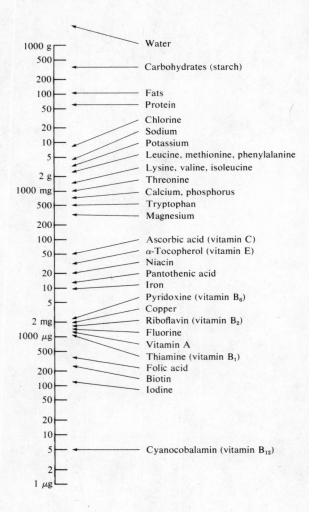

FIGURE II-1

Recommended dietary allowances for a male adult (daily intake, in foods and food supplements) of some nutrients, usually the amounts estimated as needed to prevent overt manifestation of deficiency disease in most persons. For the substances listed in smaller amounts the optimum intake, leading to the best of health, may be somewhat greater. Not shown, but probably or possibly required, are the essential fatty acids, p-aminobenzoic acid, choline, vitamin D, vitamin K, chromium, manganese, cobalt, nickel, zinc, selenium, molybdenum, vanadium, tin, and silicon.

It must be kept in mind that any person may have a special need for some nutrient, which may be then provided as a nutritional supplement. The general problem of finding the nutritional needs of a particular person has not yet been solved. Analysis of the blood, urine, or hair in some cases indicates in a reliable way the need for an increased or decreased intake of a nutrient, but often the need exists even when the measured concentration is in the "normal" range. It is impossible to get completely reliable advice about nutrition, in part because of the deficiencies in the existing methods of determining the nutritional needs of an individual, in part because of the incomplete development of nutritional science, and in part because of the lack of knowledge of the present state of the science by many physicians and nutritionists.

The value indicated in Figure II-1 for the daily intake of protein by an adult male is about 60 grams per day. This intake is somewhat larger than the amount needed to prevent protein starvation. Unless the protein is lacking in some of the essential amino acids, as it may be on an extreme vegetarian diet, or unless the person has a genetic abnormality, it would provide at least the recommended values of these essential substances, which are leucine, methionine, phenylalanine, lysine, valine, isoleucine, threonine, and tryptophan. Normal human beings are able to synthesize the other amino acids.

Vitamins are organic compounds (compounds of carbon) that occur naturally in foods and that are required in small amounts for good health. The discovery of vitamins was made gradually, over a period of centuries. It was recognized long ago that diseases such as scurvy, beriberi, rickets, and night blindness are related to the diet. Ancient Greek, Roman, and Arab physicians knew that including animal liver in the diet would prevent or cure night blindness.

The nature of the vitamins was discovered only rather recently. In the article on scurvy in the 11th edition of the Encyclopedia Britannica, published in 1911, the statement is made that the incidence of scurvy depends upon the nature of the food, but that it was not yet known with certainty whether scurvy is caused by the absence of certain constituents from the food or by the presence of some actual poison in the food. But in 1889 it had been shown by a young Dutch physician, Christiaan Eijkman, that a disease of chickens closely resembling beriberi resulted from their being fed polished rice, rather than unpolished rice, and that the chickens could be cured by adding rice polishings to their diet. He also showed that human beings did not suffer from beriberi if they ate unpolished rice rather than polished rice. Other investigators, especially the English biochemist F. Gowland Hopkins, made similar studies during the early years of the 20th century. In 1911 Casimir Funk, a Polish biochemist, published his theory of "vitamines." He suggested that four important substances are present in natural foods, providing protection against the four diseases beriberi, scurvy, pellagra, and rickets. He coined the word vitamine from the Latin word *vita,* life, and the chemical term *amine,* a member of a class of compounds of nitrogen. It was found later that some of these substances do not contain nitrogen, and the word was changed to vitamin.

The principal vitamins for human beings are vitamin A, thiamine (vitamin B1), riboflavin (vitamin B2), pyridoxine (vitamin B6), cobalamin (vitamin B12), nicotinic acid or nicotinamide (the pellagra-preventive factor), pantothenic acid, folic acid, vitamin C (L-ascorbic acid, sodium ascorbate), vitamin D (calciferol), vitamin E (the tocopherols), vitamin K, and the essential amino acids.

Appendix III

Some Information about Anticancer Drugs

As was mentioned in Chapter 7, the drugs used against cancer may be conveniently grouped into several classes, the most important being the alkylating agents, the antimetabolites, and the mitotic inhibitors.

THE ALKYLATING AGENTS

Mustard Gas (Sulfur Mustard). Too toxic to be employed in any therapeutic role.

Nitrogen Mustard (HN$_2$, Mustargen, Mechlorethamine, Mustine). A less toxic close chemical relative of the above. An alkylating agent capable of binding two adjacent guanine bases on two strands of the DNA chain, arresting cell division. Also many other cytotoxic effects throughout the cell proliferative cycle. Highly poisonous and extremely corrosive, with a very short life in the tissues. The original cytotoxic agent developed for clinical use. Of some use in almost all cancers, but particularly in the rapidly proliferating neoplasms such as the acute leukemias and malignancies of the lymphoreticular system. In quite minute doses it is an extremely powerful and indiscriminate poison affecting every kind of dividing tissue. Because of its very rapid action, of clinical value in many emergency situations such as superior vena cava compression in lung and mediastinal carcinomas. Also highly toxic to almost any other rapidly proliferating tissue.

Phenylalanine Mustard (Alkeran, Melphalan, Merphalan). In general like the above. Introduced in Britain and the USSR in the early 1950s in the hope that the incorporation of the amino acid phenylalanine, which is required in very large amounts by dividing tumor cells, would selectively increase its local concentration in tumor tissue. This is not so, but the compound appears to be particularly helpful in the management of multiple myeloma, and less so in carcinoma of the ovary and seminoma of the testis. It can be taken by mouth: bone marrow suppression appears to be the most prominent systemic toxic effect.

Cyclophosphamide (Endoxan, Cytoxan). Another alkylating agent, synthesized in Germany, and designed with the hope that it would be activated in the body only at the site of tumor-specific enzymes. The compound is metabolized in the liver with the distribution of its active agents throughout the body. Nevertheless, in practice this compound has proved to be a very valuable cytotoxic drug, and it has been used in the treatment of almost every form of cancer. It seems to have particular value in the lymphomas, in multiple myeloma, and in cancer of the breast, lung, and ovary. It is less toxic than nitrogen mustard and can be taken by mouth. In particular, it has been claimed that cyclophosphamide carries less risk of platelet suppression and bone-marrow changes in general, but it appears to carry a higher risk of alopecia (loss of hair).

Chlorambucil (Leukeran). A British product, apparently particularly toxic to lymphoid tissues and even to mature circulating lymphocytes, accounting for its considerable clinical value in the treatment of lymphomas and chronic lymphatic leukemias. From this one can judge that bone-marrow toxicity would be its specific limiting toxicity, and this is indeed so.

Busulfan (Myleran). Yet another bivalent alkylating agent, incorporating two reactive sulfur atoms in its structure. It appears to be selectively cytotoxic to granulocytes, and therefore its main clinical use is confined to the treatment of chronic myeloid (granulocytic) leukemia. As might be expected, bone-marrow suppression is the principal toxic effect.

Triethylenethiophosphoramide (Thio-Tepa, TSPA). A protein-cross-linking trivalent alkylating agent originally developed in the natural fiber textile industry. Not particularly effective, but on the other hand not particularly toxic, and can be safely instilled into natural body cavities such as the pleura and the peritoneum to retard progressive malignant colonization, and clinically to reduce malignant pleural effusions and malignant ascites in such sites. It has a relatively mild depressant effect on the bone marrow.

Ethoglucid (Epodyl). A diepoxide, again developed in the textile industry because of its specific ability to cross-link protein molecules, but with the additional special property of being able to diffuse through the blood-brain barrier. Rarely used now, but some successes in the retardation of brain tumors have been reported.

Dibromomannitol (DBM, Myelobromal). A bivalent cross-linking agent used in treating lymphomas, chronic lymphatic leukemias, and some others.

THE ANTIMETABOLITES

Methotrexate (MX, Amethopterin). This is a folic acid antagonist. All dividing cells require a regular supply of the vitamin folic acid, processed
through various enzymatic processes to its ultimate cellular nutrient, folinic
acid. If the environment of the cells is swamped by the folinic acid analog
methotrexate, they will preferentially accept the substitute, and thus be
damaged. This would be highly specific anticancer chemotherapy, were it
not for the fact that non-neoplastic normal cells are damaged in the same
way. Nevertheless, methotrexate remains high on the list of useful anticancer agents. It is possible to blast almost all of the dividing cells out of
existence by swamping them with the useless analog methotrexate, and then
to rescue the survivors (hoped to be the normal cells) by bathing them in
folic acid or, preferably, folinic acid. Although MX acts through a totally
different mechanism from the alkylating agents, the overall effects are the
same—they are quite non-specific in the sense that they interfere with the
division of any cell, whether it be normal or malignant. The major field of
usefulness of methotrexate is in the control of malignant disorders of the
blood-forming system, such as the leukemias, and, as might be expected,
their greatest toxicity is apparent in the same system.

5-Fluorouracil (5-FU). Uracil, an important part of ribonucleic acid, is selectively utilized by almost every malignant tumor. Replacing the number-5
hydrogen atom with a fluorine atom to form 5-FU creates a most effective
antimetabolite, and in practice this compound has been shown to exert an
effective cytotoxic action. For reasons not completely understood, it
appears to exert its greatest cytotoxic action against malignancies of the
gastrointestinal tract, but as might be expected its major toxicity is focused
on the gut. It has also been shown to have some value in other forms of
cancer, such as cancer of the breast, and it is also appreciably toxic to the
bone marrow.

6-Mercaptopurine (6-MP, Purinethol). This is yet another synthetic analog,
this time designed to block purine synthesis. It is useful in the maintenance
therapy of leukemias, once remission has been induced by a more potent
agent. It exerts appreciable marrow and gut toxicity, and must be prescribed
with knowledgeable caution. Because of its special mode of action, it can
produce dangerously high levels of serum uric acid with a danger of renal
failure. The anti-hyperuricemic drug allopurinol, although of no known
anticancer effect, is of value as a potentiator of 6-MP by reducing the risk of
this complication.

6-Azauridine triacetate (Azaribine). Another antagonist for nucleic acid
synthesis, used in the treatment of choriocarcinoma and mycosis fungoides.

Cytosine arabinoside (Ara-C, Cytarabine, Cytosar). Another antagonist of nucleic acid synthesis. Used in the treatment of acute granulocytic and lymphocytic leukemia.

Thioguanine (TTG). Another nucleic acid antagonist, also used in the treatment of acute leukemia.

THE ANTIMITOTIC VINCA ALKALOIDS

These alkaloids are complex nitrogenous substances of botanical origin, and the discovery of their value in cancer management was quite fortuitous. Caribbean folklore claimed that infusions from the leaves of the common garden periwinkle, *Vinca rosea,* were of some value in the control of diabetes. Eventually these claims were tested in Canada and found to be unfounded, but, far most important, the extracts were shown to exert a marked antimitotic effect. Eventually two relatively pure potent alkaloids were obtained, differing little in structure but more in pharmacological effect. These are the following:

Vincristine (Oncovin). A useful drug in combined regimes for the control of leukemias, lymphomas, and Hodgkin's disease, and, because of its special lack of marrow toxicity, a useful agent in the retardation of many other forms of cancer. The most prominent side-effect of Vincristine is irreversible damage to the brain and central nervous system, leading from peripheral neuropathy through paralysis to coma and death.

Vinblastine (Velban, Velbe). Far less neurotoxic, but far more toxic to the bone marrow. Nevertheless of restricted usefulness in the retardation of lymphomas and Hodgkin's disease, but must be used in combined regimes for maximum effect.

THE ANTIMITOTIC ANTIBIOTICS

In search for antimicrobial antibiotics from bacteria and fungi, a few compounds have been discovered that are highly poisonous to higher organisms, including man. In a few of these the range between antimitotic activity and systemic poisoning has been just sufficiently wide to permit their cautious introduction into cancer chemotherapy. Among the many hundreds of such compounds surveyed, a few have stood the test of time and are now in clinical use.

Actinomycin D. Discovered in the 1940s. Said to be of particular value in the management of three rather rare tumors, Wilms' tumor of the kidney in children, choriocarcinoma, and testicular tumor. A highly toxic compound with severe side-effects on the bone marrow, the gastrointestinal tract, and the skin.

Mitomycin C. Developed in Japan. Also extremely toxic, but said to be of some value in the retardation of gastrointestinal carcinoma.

Adriamycin (Doxorubicin). Of proven value in the treatment of many types of tumor, especially cancer of the breast and various soft tissue sarcomas. But severely toxic to bone marrow, gastrointestinal tract, and other tissues.

Bleomycin. Appears to be of particular value in squamous-cell carcinomas, and unique in that it appears to have practically no marrow toxicity. It is particularly toxic to skin and the gastrointestinal tract, and can cause fatal pulmonary fibrosis if used injudiciously.

OTHER ANTICANCER DRUGS

L-Asparaginase. Theoretically the perfect anticancer drug, exploiting one clear biochemical dissimilarity between normal and malignant cells, the inability of the latter to synthesize the amino acid asparagine. In theory, asparaginase would destroy all free asparagine and the tumor cells would die. Unfortunately, quite disappointing in clinical practice, and highly toxic to the liver. Of very limited use.

The Nitrosureas (BCNU and CCNU). Powerful cytotoxics with one advantage, that they can pass the blood-brain barrier. Have been employed with some success in brain tumors as well as other cancers. Demonstrate all the usual toxicities.

Procarbazine (MIH, Natulan). Useful in combined regimes, particularly in the management of Hodgkin's disease. Frequently produces nausea and is also mildly toxic to the bone marrow. Has the chemical structure of an antidepressant and may lead to drowsiness and mental confusion.

Cis(II)Platinum (DDP, cis-dichlorodiammineplatinum(II)). One of the newer anticancer drugs. Appears to have special value in testicular, ovarian, and bladder cancer. In addition to the usual limiting toxicities, appears to be especially toxic to the kidney, although this can be reduced by maintaining a particularly high urine output, usually by fast intravenous fluid infusion.

Appendix IV

Practical Information about Vitamin C and its Use

Vitamin C, L-ascorbic acid, is a rather simple substance, its chemical formula being $C_6H_8O_6$. It is closely related to the carbohydrates; indeed, in the cells of plants and most animals (with man being an exception) it is made from the simple sugar glucose (dextrose, grape sugar, corn sugar), which has the formula $C_6H_{12}O_6$. Ascorbic acid is a weak acid, with acid strength between that of citric acid, the principal acid in citrus fruits, and acetic acid, the acid of vinegar. It is also a chemical reducing agent, capable of combining with oxygen and serving as an antioxidant. As an antioxidant it is effective, together with vitamin E, in protecting cell membranes against damage by oxidation. In addition to this function and its function in the synthesis of collagen, it is involved in many other biochemical processes in the human body. As has been mentioned in Chapter 16, it is a very innocuous substance, essentially without serious side effects.

Ascorbic acid is prepared synthetically or extracted from fruit and vegetable sources. It should be noted that the steps used in the synthetic process are closely similar to those taking place in nature, and that there is no difference between the synthetic and the "natural" product other than the cost and possibly some impurities in the latter.

Pure ascorbic acid is a white, almost odorless crystalline powder with a sharp acidic taste. It is freely soluble in water and less so in alcohol. A 2-percent solution in water has a pH of 2.56. Aqueous solutions are somewhat unstable and tend to undergo oxidation by reacting with atmospheric oxygen, and this change is accelerated by light and by heat. Under ordinary conditions the vitamin in solution in a bottle that is kept stoppered does not oxidize very much in a week or two. The dry crystalline powder and tablets kept in a closed container are perfectly stable and have a long shelf life.

Salts of ascorbic acid are known as ascorbates, and of these sodium ascorbate and calcium ascorbate are in common use. These ascorbates have the same biological action as ascorbic acid. They are white, almost odorless fine crystalline powders. Both sodium and calcium ascorbate are freely soluble in water. Sodium ascorbate is almost tasteless, whereas the calcium salt has a brackish taste. Their aqueous solutions have a pH of around 7.8, and are thus slightly alkaline.

It should be noted that ascorbates are usually sold as ascorbic acid equivalents; that is, a 1000-mg tablet of sodium ascorbate actually contains 1125 mg of the sodium salt, and a tablet described as 1000-mg calcium ascorbate contains 1108 mg of that salt. Sodium ascorbate contains one sodium ion per ascorbate ion; calcium ascorbate contains one calcium ion for every two ascorbate ions.

Ascorbic acid and the ascorbates are marketed in the form of the pure crystalline powders, or as compressed tablets, timed-release capsules, and effervescent tablets. The powders are the cheapest and most convenient method of purchase; a kilogram (2.2 pounds) of ascorbic acid can be purchased retail for $13.25 (Bronson Pharmaceuticals, 4526 Rinetti Lane, La Canada, California 91011). One level teaspoon of the powder is approximately 4.5 grams. The tablets are available in a variety of sizes: 50 mg, 100 mg, 250 mg, 500 mg and 1 gram (1000 mg). The timed-release capsules may avoid gastrointestinal upset and are believed by some to be of special value in dealing with colonic disease. Effervescent tablets contain ascorbic acid and sodium bicarbonate, which react in water to produce a very refreshing drink, but they are a somewhat expensive way to acquire large amounts of vitamin C. A palatable effervescent drink can be made by putting one level teaspoonful of ascorbic acid in water and adding ¼ to ½ as much baking soda (sodium hydrogen carbonate).

Ascorbic acid or ascorbate crystals may be taken mixed in water or fruit juice. In the original trials with far advanced cancer patients in Vale of Leven Hospital a somewhat old-fashioned formula was devised:

Ascorbic acid	100 grams
Sodium bicarbonate	48 grams
70% Sorbitol syrup	200 milliliters
Distilled water to	600 milliliters

Take 15 ml (1 tablespoon = 2.5 grams sodium ascorbate) four times a day after meals. The mixture to be continued indefinitely.

This mixture, devised for far-advanced patients, has proved to be very popular in general use. The disadvantage is that it must be dispensed in dark bottles and preferably be stored in the refrigerator because of its limited shelf life (about four weeks).

The dose of oral vitamin C to obtain the maximum benefit in cancer has still to be determined, but the indications are that the requirement is roughly related to the extent of the disease, which in turn is the product of the extent of the tumor multiplied by its rate of growth. Thus the requirement for a small slowly growing tumor will be very much less than for a rapidly growing widely disseminated lesion. There are good clinical grounds for the belief, first expounded by Dr. Robert Cathcart, that bowel tolerance gives a fairly reliable indication of requirement. Our general recommendation for cancer patients would be to start at 1 g per day, and increase the daily intake by 1 g on each subsequent day, in divided doses, until diarrhea develops, then reduce the dose by 1 g below this tolerance dose and maintain that dose indefinitely thereafter.

In certain circumstances, vitamin C cannot be taken by mouth and has to be given by the physician or surgeon by injection. Injectable vitamin C is prepared in sterile ampoules in the form of sodium ascorbate. Sources known to us are the following:

Size	Content as ascorbic acid equivalent	Supplier
2 ml	500 mg	Vitarin Co., Ltd. 227-15 North Conduit Avenue Springfield Gardens, N.Y. 11413
30 ml	7,500 mg	Bronson Pharmaceuticals 4526 Rinetti Lane La Canada, California 91011
20 ml	4,000 mg	
30 ml	7,500 mg	Fellows Medical Mfg. Co. Oak Park, Michigan 48237

The contents of these ampoules can be given by deep intramuscular injection, but the procedure is painful and not to be recommended. Intravenous administration is preferable.

Ascorbate can be injected intravenously as a "one-shot" procedure, but for prolonged course the continuous intravenous infusion of a sodium ascorbate solution is preferable. To reduce the risk of chemical phlebitis in the receiving vein, we prefer to use a long-line caval catheter such as the "E-Z Cath" manufactured by C. R. Bard. The catheter is introduced in the usual fashion through a peripheral vein on the front of the elbow and the tip is advanced until it lies within the main veins of the thorax. For a carrier solution we prefer to use Ringer's lactate given at an infusion rate of 2 liters per day. The ampoules of sodium ascorbate are added to the flasks of Ringer's lactate solution under full aseptic precautions.

We emphasize the importance of continued administration of ascorbic acid or ascorbate. It should not be stopped for even a single day (see Chapter 16, the rebound effect), except possibly during the administration of a chemotherapeutic agent, as suggested in Chapter 23.

Appendix V

A Discussion
of Surgical Terms

Many patients find the working language of surgeons highly confusing, and yet its structure follows a few simple rules. To describe any surgical operation, the organ operated upon is first identified by its Latin root, followed by a suffix describing the operative procedure. In operative situations where two or more organs are involved, accepted style requires that the organs be listed in the "direction of flow," as, for instance, stomach to intestine, intestine to colon, ureter to bladder, and womb to fallopian tube to ovary. Because the number of individual surgical procedures that can be performed is limited, the suffixes we have to consider are few. The following examples may serve to clarify the situation:

-centesis: the withdrawal of an abnormal accumulation of fluid from a body cavity. Examples are *thoracocentesis,* the aspiration of a pleural effusion; *paracentesis* (more correctly, paracentesis abdominis), the aspiration from the abdominal cavity of an abnormal collection of fluid, known as ascites; *pericardiocentesis,* the aspiration of fluid from within the pericardial sac surrounding the heart.

-ectomy: the cutting out of, or the excision of. These operations are often subdivided according to their extent into such categories as partial, subtotal, total, and radical, the last implying the concurrent removal of all adjacent lymph nodes, with, in certain circumstances, even an extra category, supraradical, meaning the additional removal of lymph nodes not in the immediate surgical field. Some common examples are *hypophysectomy,* the removal of the pituitary gland; *thyroidectomy,* the removal of the thyroid gland; *mastectomy,* the removal of the breast; *esophagectomy,* the removal of a diseased segment of the esophagus; *lobectomy,* removal of a diseased lung lobe; *pneumonectomy,* removal of a whole diseased lung; *gastrectomy,* removal of the stomach; *enterectomy,* the removal of a diseased segment of small intestine; *colectomy,* the removal of a diseased segment of the large intestine; *prostatectomy,* the removal of the prostate gland; *cystectomy,* the removal of the urinary bladder; *nephrectomy,* the removal of a kidney;

212

cholecystectomy, the removal of the gallbladder; *splenectomy*, the removal of the spleen; *pancreatectomy*, the removal of the pancreas; with such obvious variants as *total cysto-prostatectomy*, the removal of the whole urinary bladder and the prostate gland, usually for bladder-based cancer, and *hystero-salpingo-oophorectomy*, the removal of the uterus, both fallopian tubes, and both ovaries. A *Wertheim's hysterectomy* is an extension of the above to include the careful removal of all pelvic lymph nodes. An *abdomino-perineal excision of the rectum* describes removal of the lower sigmoid colon, the rectum, and the anus for rectal cancer. In the case of paired organs, such as the ovaries, the testes, or the adrenal glands, where both organs of the pair are removed the operations are described as *bilateral oophorectomies, bilateral orchidectomies,* and *bilateral adrenalectomies,* respectively.

-graphy: the detection and usually the recording of abnormalities by physical means. The simplest example is *clinical photography* where, say, the size of an expanding skin lesion is recorded by serial photographs. *Radiography*, obtaining pictures by the use of x-rays, is invaluable for the study and recording of changes in internal structures. *Plain radiography* is based upon the varying translucencies of different tissue to x-ray penetration as observed on a fluorescent screen or recorded on a photographic film; in this way it is easy to see the distinction between a normal translucent aerated lung and a dense tumor or a normal skeletal structure and a metastasis. To improve the definition of deeper structures, *tomography* is sometimes used; in this technique, the x-ray source and the x-ray plate are pivoted in opposing directions during exposure, producing a sharp image of the pivotal point, and blurring of other layers. A comparatively recent and highly technical innovation has been the introduction of *computerized axial tomography* (the so-called CAT-scan, or EMI-scan). In this technique the source of a thin beam of x-rays is continually rotated around the patient to be picked up by a sensitive detector rotating synchronously always at the opposite point in the equatorial plane. By the use of computer technology, this signal is translated to produce very detailed pictures of complete cross-sections or "slices" of the body. In this way the detailed outline and structure of many internal organs not readily accessible to routine radiography can be obtained.

Mammography is the use of low-penetration x-rays to obtain a gray-upon-gray contrasting image of the intrinsic structure of the human breast. There is no doubt that this technique can recognize with a fair degree of accuracy many early breast cancers. One problem is that routine mammography involving cumulative doses of carcinogenic irradiation might cause more cancers than it detects. *Contrast radiography* describes the use of some intensely radio-opaque substance to outline the contour and motility of some internal organ, and by demonstrating some focal point of abnormality indicate with a high degree of accuracy the correct diagnosis. The contrast substance may be non-absorbable barium sulfate suspensions, either swallowed or given by enema to demonstrate abnormalities of the upper or lower alimentary tract, respectively. Both types of examination may be combined into what has come to be known as "a full G.I. series" to study the whole gastrointestinal tract, usually for cancer.

To obtain diagnostic information about the conformation of less accessible organs, we have to employ special radio-opaque compounds which given either orally or intravenously tend to be concentrated in the target organ. Among the former are compounds that tend to be excreted in the bile *(oral cholecystography, intravenous cholangiography)*, which can depict the gallbladder, or the gallbladder and bile ducts, respectively. Somewhat similar compounds given intravenously are selectively excreted in the urine and can produce excellent pictures of kidney, ureter, and bladder structure *(intravenous* or *descending pyelography)*. In certain anatomical situations it is necessary to inject the radio-opaque substance directly into the body space we wish to visualize. One long established technique is the injection of sodium iodide by cystoscope through a ureteric catheter to obtain a very sharp outline of the kidney's collecting system *(a retrograde* or *ascending pyelogram)*. By simplifying the technique, we can obtain a *retrograde cystogram* outlining the urinary bladder to demonstrate, for instance, any tumor within. *Myelography* describes the injection of radio-opaque materials into the spinal canal. An extension of these techniques, requiring considerable expertise, is selective *angiography (arteriography)*. In these procedures, a very long and very fine plastic tube (a catheter) is carefully manipulated under x-ray guidance into the main artery of the target organ. Once precisely located, a brisk injection of the radio-opaque material followed almost instantaneously by a radiograph will demonstrate the vascular structure. In the case of the kidney, for example, an absence of vascularity will almost certainly indicate a cyst, whereas a profusion of vascularity will be strong evidence of a tumor.

Lymphangiography, a technique also requiring considerable expertise, is the injection of radio-opaque dyes into lymphatics to outline lymph nodes and to ascertain whether or not they are free of malignant involvement. In certain circumstances, instead of using radio-opaque materials better contrast and definition can be obtained by using a radio-translucent substance such as air. Thus in *air encephalography*, the carefully controlled introduction of air into the spinal cavity, the air will rise and outline the surface of the brain within the skull. Air can also be used to separate and outline the individual structures in the mediastinum *(mediastinography)*.

The relative increased vascularity of cancers has given rise to the employment of a number of other physical methods in diagnosis. The simplest of these is *thermography*, in which an infrared heat recording camera is used. If we stand a healthy young woman before such a camera, the record will only show a uniform glow, but if she has a nascent breast cancer the picture will be marred by one localized hot spot, indicating the tumor.

For the visualization of increased vascularity in deeper structures we have to employ radioactive isotopes that tend to be localized in the tissue to be studied, and then record the resulting radiation emission using a sensitive gamma-ray camera. The two applications of this technique in common use are the so-called liver scan and the bone scan. In the former, after the administration of the suitable compound the radioactivity of the liver is scanned linearly, as in a television picture. A healthy liver will produce a smooth picture of uniform density; in contrast, liver metastases produce an irregular fragmented picture, with the degree of irregularity proportional to the extent of malignant involvement. In the bone scan a picture of the whole skeleton is obtained with points of skeletal metastases showing up as local hot spots of increasing density. It should be noted that some skeletal metastases invisible on plain radiography may be demonstrated by bone scan, but that some skeletal metastases clearly visible on plain x-ray photographs may fail to be detected by bone scan.

The last physical agent to be routinely used in diagnostic investigation is *ultrasonography*, the use of high-frequency sound waves developed from the war-time invention of Sonar. Electronic means are used to separate the reflected echoes into coherent pictures. In effect, this technique measures boundaries, the edges of individual organs, and changes in structure within the tissues of individual organs. In cancer, it is of particular value in distinguishing between true and false tumors (such as cysts) and, at a more sophisticated level, identifying and measuring with a fair degree of accuracy the presence and size of metastases in soft tissue organs such as the liver.

-ology: knowledge about the particular subject; **-ologist:** one who professes to have acquired special knowledge about the particular subject. Familiar examples are *biology*, an understanding of fundamental life processes; *cardiology*, an understanding of the heart; *cytology*, an understanding of cell structure and function (but a *cytologist* is a person skilled in detecting the characteristics of malignant cells); *gastroenterology*, an understanding of the whole alimentary tract and its related secretory organs; *histology* (or *histopathology*), an understanding of the microscopic appearances of different tissues; *immunology*, an understanding of the immune processes that protect the individual against extraneous assault; *nephrology*, an understanding of functional disease of the kidney; *oncology*, an understanding of the unique properties of cancer cells (but current usage of the term *oncologist* has come to mean narrow expertise in the use of cancer chemotherapeutic drugs); *psychology*, an understanding of the workings of the human mind (as opposed to *neurology*, the "mechanistic" approach, which importantly relates defects in function to defects in neuro-muscular transmission); *respiratology*, the understanding of the whole oxygenation system; *trauma-*

tology, an understanding of the effects of injury; *urology*, an understanding of any abnormalities of the urogenital tract; *zoology*, an understanding of features of animal structure, function, and behavior.

-orrhaphy: the repair of some defect. An example is *herniorrhaphy*, the repair of a hernial defect.

-oscopy: the visual examination of the interior of some body cavity or organ. Such examinations require the use of some specially designed instrument incorporating a light source to illuminate the cavity and an optical system for the visualization of the contents. The original instruments were of rigid construction with classical lenses and prisms and with obvious mechanical difficulties and restrictions on their use. Modern fiberoptic technology has led to the design of soft flexible instruments that can negotiate sharp contours and still present a clear visual image. Some common examples are *laparoscopy*, visual examination of the contents of the abdominal cavity; *bronchoscopy*, visual examination of the bronchial tree; *cystoscopy*, visual inspection of the bladder interior and contents; *proctoscopy*, visual examination of the rectum; *sigmoidoscopy*, inspection of the interior of the rectum and lower sigmoid colon; *coloscopy*, examination (usually under high magnification) of the surface of the uterine cervix; *gastroscopy* and *esophagoscopy*, examination of the lining of the upper alimentary tract; and the compendium word, *endoscopy*, which strictly speaking includes all such examinations but in practice has come to be limited to visual examination of the upper alimentary tract; it is, in fact, *esophago-gastro-duodenoscopy*. If any operative procedures are carried out through such instruments, such operations are prefaced by the appropriate adjective. Common examples are *laparascopic sterilization, bronchoscopic biopsy, cystoscopic ureteral catheterization, colonoscopic or gastroscopic polypectomy*.

-ostomy: the formation of a permanent or semipermanent opening or channel. If the opening is onto the skin, only the underlying organ need be mentioned. Common examples are *tracheostomy*, an opening into the trachea to relieve respiratory obstruction; *gastrostomy*, an opening into the stomach for nutrients to relieve esophageal obstruction; *colostomy*, an emergency opening into the colon to relieve large bowel obstruction or as a permanent feature after removal of the distal colon; *nephrostomy*, an opening into the kidney, or *ureterostomy*, an opening into the ureter, in both cases, an opening onto the skin to relieve lower urinary tract obstruction. If such a channel is surgically created internally between two organs, convention decrees that such operations always be described in "the direction of the flow" qualified by the same suffix. Common examples are: *gastroenterostomy*, the formation of a passage between the interior of the stomach and the interior of the small intestine; an *ileo-transverse colostomy*, the surgical formation of a channel between the distal small intestine and the transverse colon; *cecocolostomy*, the formation of a channel between the cecum and somewhere farther along the colon; *ureterosigmoidostomy*, surgical connection to enable the ureters to drain into the sigmoid colon to by-pass an obstructed bladder, usually caused by cancer. The words *cholecystogastrostomy*, *cholecystojejunostomy*, *choledochoduodenostomy*, and *hepaticoduodenostomy* describe operations to relieve bile duct obstruction, usually because of pancreatic cancer, allowing bile to drain into the alimentary tract, by-passing the tumor.

-otomy: the cutting into or the cutting across. Examples of cutting into are *laparotomy*, an exploratory opening into the abdominal cavity; *thoracotomy*, an exploratory incision into the thoracic cavity (the chest); *craniotomy*, an exploratory opening into the skull; *arthrotomy;* an exploratory opening into a joint; *arteriotomy*, an exploratory opening into an artery; and *phlebotomy*, an exploratory opening into a vein. Examples of cutting across are *osteotomy*, the cutting across of a bone, usually to correct malalignment; *vagotomy*, the cutting across of the vagal nerves to reduce secretion of gastric acid and pepsin; *lobotomy*, the cutting across of nerve fibers from a lobe of the brain, usually the frontal lobe, to attempt to reduce, in that instance, abnormal psychiatric stimuli; and *chordotomy*, the selective division of certain tracts in the spinal cord for the relief of pain.

-pexy: the fixation of an abnormally mobile organ. Examples are *nephropexy*, fixation of an abnormally mobile kidney; *gastropexy*, fixation of an abnormally mobile stomach; and *cecopexy*, fixation of an abnormally mobile cecum.

-plasty: the refashioning of to form a more acceptable or better functioning contour. Some common examples are *rhinoplasty*, a cosmetic refashioning of the shape of the nose; *pyloroplasty*, a refashioning of the pyloric canal of the stomach to facilitate better drainage from the stomach; *mammoplasty*, refashioning the contour of the breast; and *urethroplasty*, the refashioning of an abnormal urethral passage.

Glossary

Definitions of some words used in the body of this book are given here. The kinds of cancer are described in Chapter 3, the names of anticancer drugs are given in Appendix III, and surgical terms are discussed in Appendix V; these words in general are not included in this glossary.

alkylating agent: a substance that transfers alkyl groups (such as the methyl group, CH_3) to another substance, replacing a hydrogen atom.

anaplastic: lacking in differentiated structure: The reversion (of cells) to a more primitive embryonal type.

anastomosis: either a naturally-occurring communication or a surgically-created connection between two structures such as the divided ends of the intestine after resection.

anorexia: diminished appetite, aversion to food.

antibody: A blood protein (immunoglobulin) with the power of combining specifically with a molecule or group of atoms (the antigen or haptenic group).

antigen: Any molecule that has the power, when introduced into the body, of causing an animal to produce antibody molecules.

antimetabolite: a substance that competes with a metabolite and prevents it from carrying out its function.

aorta: the main artery leading from the heart, the main trunk of the arterial system.

ascites: the accumulation of fluid in the abdominal cavity.

atrophic: literally "wasted" or "shrunken." In cancer, an adjective used to describe tumors where the scarring is so intense that the surrounding tissues are contracted.

BCG: Abbreviation for bacillus of Calmette and Guerin, used as a vaccine for tuberculosis, and also as an immune stimulant in the treatment of cancer.

benign tumor: a tumor which is non-invasive and non-malignant.

bronchus: the main air passages leading from the trachea (windpipe) to the lungs.

cachexia: a feeling of misery, with malnutrition and wasting of the body, found in many patients with cancer and some other diseases.

cancer: any of the various types of malignant neoplasms, and as a general term, the illness caused by them.

carcinogen: Any cancer-producing substance or condition.

carcinogenic: Having the property of causing cancer.

carcinoma: A malignant tumor of epithelial or endothelial origin.

carcinomatosis: The condition of having widespread carcinoma involving multiple sites.

cholecystitis: Inflammation of the gall-bladder.

chromosome: A collection of genes and supporting structures in the nucleus of a cell.

clone: A colony or group of cells or organisms that have arisen by asexual reproduction from a single individual.

collagen: a fibrous protein, the major constituent of the white fibers of connective tissue, ground substance, cartilage, and bone.

collagenase: An enzyme that catalyzes the splitting of molecules of collagen into smaller molecules.

complement: A complex of blood proteins that combine with antigen-antibody complexes and assist in their destruction by lymphocytes.

cystoscopic: Relating to the inspection of the interior of the bladder with the use of a lighted optical instrument.

cytostasis: The slowing of the proliferative rate of cells.

cytotoxic: able to destroy cells.

diagnosis: the determination of the nature of a disease.

DNA, deoxyribonucleic acid: the self-replicating substance of genes and many viruses.

encapsulation: the enclosure within a capsule of fibrous tissue.

endocarditis: inflammation of the endocardium, the lining membrane of the heart and heart valves.

endotoxic: containing bacterial toxins that are not freely liberated into the surrounding medium.

enzyme: a protein secreted by cells that acts as a catalyst to increase the rate of a chemical reaction, without itself being changed.

epithelium: an outer layer of cells covering the skin and other surfaces.

erythrocyte: a red blood cell (red corpuscle).

erysipelas: an acute febrile illness arising from spreading hemolytic strepto-coccal infection of the skin.

erythrocyte sedimentation rate: the rate at which red blood cells fall toward the bottom of a tube, a measure of the severity of illness.

exogenous: originating or produced outside.

fibroblast: an elongated cell present in connective tissue and capable of forming collagen fibrils.

fibroid: resembling fibrous tissue. Wrongly but by common usage, a descrip-tive term for a benign myoma of the uterus.

gene: the functioning unit of heredity, consisting of a chain of nucleotides, the units of DNA.

genetic: relating to the branch of science dealing with heredity.

glycosaminoglycan: a nitrogen-containing carbohydrate macromolecule, a principal constituent of ground substance.

ground substance: the intercellular cement, containing large molecules of glycosaminoglycans and fibrils of collagen.

hapten: The groups of atoms of an antigen with which the corresponding antibody combines.

hematuria: any condition in which the urine contains blood or red blood cells.

hemicolectomy: removal of approximately half of the colon.

hemorrhage: bleeding, a flow of blood.

hepatomegaly: a pathological enlargement of the liver.

hilar: relating to the hilus, which is the part of an organ where the blood vessels and nerves enter and leave.

homeostasis: the state of equilibrium in the body with respect to various functions and the composition of body fluids and tissues: the process by which this state of equilibrium is achieved.

iatrogenic: illness produced by a physician or medication as a result of erroneous or inadvertent treatment.

immunocompetence: the condition of having an effective immune mech-anism.

immunoglobulin: a protein in the blood with antibody activity; an antibody.

inflammation: the response of tissues to injury, infection, or abnormal stimu-lation—redness, increased temperature, swelling, pain.

jaundice: a yellowish staining of the skin and other tissues by bile pigments.

jejunum: the upper part of the small intestine, between the duodenum and the lower small intestine (the ileum).

laparotomy: A surgical incision into the abdominal cavity performed for exploratory purposes.

leukocyte (leucocyte): any one of the white blood cells—granulocytes (polymorphonuclear leucocytes) or lymphocytes.

lymph: the fluid that flows in the lymphatic system, and eventually empties into the venous circulation.

lymphatic: pertaining to lymph; a vessel that transports lymph; a lymph node.

lymph node (lymph gland): a discrete collection of lymphocytes situated at the junction of lymphatic vessels.

lymphocyte: lymph cells—white blood cells formed in lymphoid tissues throughout the body (lymph nodes, spleen, and thymus glands).

macrophage: a large cell with the ability to destroy bacteria and dead or abnormal cells.

malignant tumor: a tumor showing invasive properties.

megavitamin therapy: the treatment of disease by use of much larger amounts of vitamins than are usually ingested.

mesentery: the fan-shaped fold of the peritoneum carrying the blood supply and lymphatic drainage of the intestine.

mesothelioma: a rare form of cancer derived from the lining cells of the pleura or peritoneum, usually associated with exposure to asbestos fibers.

metabolism: the sum of the chemical reactions involved in the function of nutrition.

metabolite: a substance involved in or produced by the process of metabolism.

metastasis, pl. metastases, or secondary tumors: tumors that appear in parts of the body remote from the site of the primary tumor, as a result of blood-borne or lymphatic spread.

mitosis: cell division, the process by which one cell is converted into two daughter cells with the same chromosome and DNA content as the parent cell.

mitotic inhibitor: a substance that prevents mitosis.

mucosa (from tunica mucosa): mucous membrane.

necrosis: death of cells, tissues, or organs.

necrotic: affected by or pertaining to necrosis.

neoplasm: a new growth or tumor, either benign or malignant.

nucleotide: a structural unit of nucleic acids, such as DNA, a compound of phosphoric acid, a sugar (deoxyribose in DNA) and a purine or pyrimidine.

oophorectomy: removal of the ovaries.

orchidectomy, orchiectomy: removal of one or both testes.

orthomolecular: consisting of molecules that are normally present in the human body, usually characterized by low toxicity and freedom from serious side effects.

orthomolecular medicine: the achievement and preservation of good health and the prevention and treatment of disease by changing the concentrations of substances normally present in the human body.

osteoporosis: reduction in the mineral content of bone.

paresis: partial paralysis.

periosteum: the thick fibrous membrane covering the surface of bone.

periostitis: inflammation of the periosteum.

peritoneum: the serous lining of the abdominal cavity and covering for most of the viscera.

peritonitis: inflammation of the peritoneum.

platelet: an irregularly shaped disc in the circulating blood essential for blood-clotting.

pleura: the membrane lining the thoracic cavity and covering the adjacent surface of the lung.

precancer: a lesion which has a significant probability of developing into cancer in the course of time.

prognosis: the foretelling of the probable course of a disease.

prostaglandin: a class of physiologically active substances present in many tissues.

purulent: containing pus.

pyogenic: pus-forming.

pyrexia: fever.

regression: the progressive subsidence of a disease.

remission: a temporary lessening in the severity of a disease.

resectable: amenable to surgical removal.

resection: the surgical removal of an organ or part of an organ or tissue.

reticulo-endothelial system: the system of lymphocytes and other macrophages capable of destroying foreign cells, present in the network of the spleen, lymph nodes, and other organs.

reticulosis: a malignant disease of some part of the reticulo-endothelial system.

retrabeculation: the renewed formation of a framework of a bony structure.

scirrhous: hard, fibrous.

scrotum: the bag of skin and muscles containing the testes.

seromucoid: a complex of protein and polysaccharide found in blood serum.

serum seromucoid concentration: the concentration of seromucoid in blood serum giving a measure of the severity of an illness.

somatic: relating to cells and tissues other than genetic (those involved in the hereditary process).

Staphylococcus: a genus of bacteria that can cause food poisoning and produce toxins.

Streptococcus: a genus of bacteria that cause inflammation and produce toxins.

stroma: the framework of connective tissue of an organ, gland, or other structure, including a tumor.

thoracotomy: an operative incision opening into the chest cavity.

tissue: a collection of similar cells and the intercellular substances surrounding them.

T-lymphocyte: a lymphocyte produced by the thymus.

toxemia: clinical manifestations of some diseases believed to be caused by toxins or other noxious substances liberated into the blood.

toximolecular: consisting of molecules that exert a toxic or poisonous action, as with most drugs (in contrast to orthomolecular).

trauma: a wound or injury.

tumor: a swelling; a neoplasm.

tylectomy: an operation restricted to the local removal of a tumor.

ulcer: a lesion on the skin or mucous membrane surface, with superficial loss of tissue and usually with inflammation.

vaccine: a microbial preparation used for the prevention of disease.

vascularity: the condition of containing blood vessels.

vena cava (superior and inferior): the two large veins returning blood to the heart.

villus, pl. villi: a projection from the surface of a mucous membrane, such as the lining of the small intestine.

REFERENCES

Agran, L. (1977) *The Cancer Connection and What We Can Do About It.* Houghton Mifflin Company, Boston. 220 pages. An engrossing account of the history of some cancer patients and a telling discussion of the causes of cancer, especially cigarette smoking and industrial chemicals.

Altman, P. L., and Dittmer, D. S. (1968) *Metabolism.* Federation of American Societies for Experimental Biology, Bethesda, *Maryland.*

Anonymous (1976) *Vitamin C toxicity. Nutrition Reviews, 34:* 236–237.

Appelbaum, H. (1937) *Vitamin C und Krebskranken,* Dissertation for M.D. degree, thesis deposited with the University of Zurich.

Bartlett, M. K., Jones, C. M., and Ryan, A. E. (1942) Vitamin C and wound healing. II. Ascorbic acid content and tensile strength of healing wounds in human beings. *New England Journal of Medicine, 226:* 474–481.

Bjelke, E. (1973) Epidemiologic studies of cancer of the stomach, colon and rectum, Dissertation, University of Minnesota.

Bjelke, E. (1974) Epidemiologic studies of cancer of the stomach, colon and rectum with special emphasis on the role of diet. *Scand. J. Gastroenterology, 9* (Suppl. 31): 1–235.

Boyd, W. (1966) *The Spontaneous Regression of Cancer.* Charles C. Thomas, Springfield, Illinois.

Cairns, John. (1978) *Cancer: Science and Society.* W. H. Freeman and Company, San Francisco. 199 pages. A reliable general discussion of the cancer problem, except that vitamin C and nutrition are not mentioned.

Cameron, E. (1966) *Hyaluronidase and Cancer.* Pergamon Press, New York. 245 pages. A detailed discussion of the possibility of controlling cancer by protecting and strengthening the intercellular cement in the normal tissues.

Cameron, E. (1975) Vitamin C. *British Journal Hospital Medicine 13,* 511.

Cameron, E. (1976) Biological function of ascorbic acid and the pathogenesis of scurvy. *Medical Hypotheses 2:* 154–163.

Cameron, E., and Baird, G. (1973) Ascorbic acid and dependence on opiates in patients with advanced disseminated cancer. IRCS Letter to the Editor, August.

Cameron, E., and Campbell, A. (1974) The orthomolecular treatment of cancer. II. Clinical trial of high-dose ascorbic acid supplements in advanced human cancer. Chem.-Biol. Interact. 9: 285–315.

Cameron, E., Campbell, A., and Jack, T. (1975) The orthomolecular treatment of cancer. III. Reticulum cell sarcoma: double complete regression induced by high-dose ascorbic acid therapy. Chem.-Biol. Interact. 11: 387–393.

Cameron, E., and Pauling, L. (1973) Ascorbic acid and the glycosaminoglycans: an orthomolecular approach to cancer and other diseases. Oncology 27: 181–192.

Cameron, E., and Pauling, L. (1974) The orthomolecular treatment of cancer. I. The role of ascorbic acid in host resistance. Chem.-Biol. Interact. 9: 273–283.

Cameron, E., and Pauling, L. (1976) Supplementary ascorbate in the supportive treatment of cancer: prolongation of survival times in terminal human cancer. Proc. Natl. Acad. Sci. USA 73: 3685–3689.

Cameron, E., and Pauling L. (1978) Supplemental ascorbate in the supportive treatment of cancer: reevaluation of prolongation of survival times in terminal human cancer. Proc. Natl. Acad. Sci. USA 75: 4538–4542.

Cameron, E., and Pauling, L. (1978) Experimental studies designed to evaluate the management of patients with incurable cancer. Proc. Natl. Acad. Sci. USA 75: 6252.

Cameron, E., and Pauling L. (1979) Ascorbate and cancer. Proc. Am. Phil. Soc. 123: 117–123.

Cameron, E., and Pauling L. (1979) Ascorbic acid as a therapeutic agent in cancer. J. Internatl. Acad. Prevent. Med. 5, 8–29.

Cameron, E. and Pauling L., Survival times of terminal lung cancer patients treated with ascorbate. Proc. Interntl. Acad. Preventive Med., in press, 1979.

Cameron, E., Pauling, L. and Leibovitz, B. (1979) Ascorbic acid and cancer: a review. Cancer Research 39: 663–681.

Cameron, E., and Rotman, D. (1972) Ascorbic acid, cell proliferation, and cancer. Lancet i: 542.

Campbell, G. D., Jr., Steinberg, M. H., and Bower, J. D. (1975) Ascorbic acid-induced hemolysis in G-6-PD deficiency. Ann. Int. Med. 82: 810–815.

Cheraskin, E., Ringsdorf, W. M., Jr., Hutchins, K., Setyaadmadja, A. T. S. H. and Wideman, G. L. (1968) Effect of diet upon radiation response in cervical carcinoma of the uterus: A preliminary report. Acta Cytologica 12: 433–438.

Chope, H. D., and Breslow, L. (1955) Nutritional status of the aging. Am. J. Public Health 46: 61–67.

Crandon, J. H. (1955) Nutrition in surgical patients. J. Am. Med. Assoc. 158: 264–268.

Creagan, E. T., Moertel, C. G., O'Fallon, J. R., Schutt, A. J., O'Connell, M. J., Rubin, J., and Frytak, S. (1979) Failure of high-dose vitamin C (ascorbic acid) therapy to benefit patients with advanced cancer; a controlled trial. New England J. Med. issue of 27 September.

DeCosse, J. J., Adams, M. B., Kuzma, J. F., LoGerfo, P., and Condon, R. E. (1975) Effect of ascorbic acid on rectal polyps of patients with familial polyposis. Surgery 78: 608–612.

Demole, V. (1934) On the physiological action of ascorbic acid and some related compounds. *Biochemical Journal 28:* 770–773.

Deucher, W. G. (1940) Observations on the metabolism of vitamin C in cancer patients (in German). *Strahlentherapie 67:* 143–151.

Doll, R. (1977) *Origins of Human Cancer: Book A. Incidence of Cancer in Humans.* Eds: Hiatt, H. H., Walson, J. D. and Winsten, J. A. Cold Spring Harbor Laboratory, pages 1–12.

Dvorak, H. F., Dvorak, A. M., Manseau, E. J., Wiberg, L. and Churchill, W. H. (1979) Fibrin gel investment associated with line 1 and line 10 solid tumor growth, angiogenesis, and fibroplasia in guinea pigs. Role of cellular immunity, myofibroblasts, microvascular damage, and infarction in line 1 tumor regression. *J. Natl. Cancer Inst. 62:* 1459–1472.

Eckholm, E. P. (1977) *The Picture of Health: Environmental Sources of Disease.* W. W. Norton and Company, Inc., New York. 256 pages. A general discussion of health, environmental factors, undernutrition, and other topics, but with no mention of vitamin C.

Epstein, S. S. (1978) *The Politics of Cancer.* Sierra Club Books, San Francisco. 583 pages. A thorough study of the cancer problem with emphasis on the actions of industries and of government agencies in causing and controlling the disease and the strong recommendation that great efforts to prevent cancer are needed. A brief discussion of vitamin C is included.

Everson, T. C., and Cole, W. H. (1966) *Spontaneous Repression of Cancer.* A study and abstract of reports in the world medical literature and of personal communications concerning spontaneous regression of malignant disease. W. B. Saunders Company, Philadelphia.

Gerson, M. (1958) *A Cancer Therapy: Results of Fifty Cases.* Totality Books, Del Mar, California, 2nd edition. 432 pages.

Harris, A., Robinson, A. B., and Pauling L. Blood plasma L-ascorbic acid concentration for oral L-ascorbic acid dosage up to 12 grams per day. *International Research Communications System,* page 19, December, 1973.

Hines, K., and Danes, B. H. (1976) Microtubular defect in Chediak-Higashi syndrome. *Lancet,* 145–146, 17 July.

Horrobin, D., Manku, M. S., Oka, M., Morgan, R. O., Cunnane, S. C., Ally, A. I., Zhayur, T., Schweitzer, M., and Karmali, R. A. (1979) The nutritional regulation of T-lymphocyte function. *Med. Hypotheses 5:* 969–985.

Horrobin, D. F., Oka, M., and Manku, M. S. (1979) The regulation of prostaglandin E1 formation: a candidate for one of the fundamental mechanisms involved in the actions of vitamin C. *Med. Hypotheses 5:* 849–858.

Jones, H. B. (1956) Demographic consideration of the cancer problem. *Trans. N. Y. Acad. Sci. 18:* 298–333.

Klenner, F. R. (1951) Massive doses of vitamin C and the viral diseases. *Southn. Med. & Surg. 113:* 101–107.

Klenner, R. F. (1971) Observations on the dose and administration of ascorbic acid when employed beyond the range of a vitamin in human pathology. *J. Appl. Nutr. 23:* 61–88.

Lai, H-Y L., Shields, Eleanor K. and Watne, A. L. (1977) Effect of ascorbic acid on rectal polyps and fecal steroids. *Fed. Proc.* (Abs.) *35:* 1061.

Libby, A. F., and Stone I. (1977) The hypoascorbemia-kwashiorkor approach to drug addiction therapy: A pilot study. *J. Orthomolecular Psychiatry, 6:* 300–308.

Lind, J. (1753) A treatise on the scurvy. Edinburgh: Sands, Murray and Cochrane. Reprinted C. P. Stewart and D. Guthrie (eds). Edinburgh: Edinburgh University Press, 1953.

McCann, J., and Ames, B. N. (1977) The Salmonella/*typhimurium* microsome mutagenicity test: Predictive value for animal carcinogenicity, pp. 1431 to 1450 in *Origins of Human Cancer: Book C, Human Risk Assessment.* Eds: Hiatt, H. H., Watson, J. D. and Winston, J. A. Cold Spring Harbor Laboratory.

McPherson, K., and Fox, M. S. (1977) Treatment of breast cancer. pp. 308 to 322 in *Costs, Risks, and Benefits of Surgery.* Eds: Bunker, J. P., Barnes, B. A. and Mosteller, F. New York: Oxford University Press.

McWhirter, R. (1948) The value of simple mastectomy and radiotherapy in the treatment of cancer of the breast. *Brit. J. Radiol. 21:* 252.

Miller, N. E., Forde, O. H., Thelle, D. S. and Mjos, O. D. (1977) The Tromso heart study: high density liproprotein and coronary heart disease, a prospective case-control study. *Lancet i:* 965.

Moertel, S. G. (1978) Current concepts in cancer: chemotherapy of gastrointestinal cancer. *New Engl. J. Med. 299:* 1049–1052.

Morishige, F., and Murata, A. (1978) Vitamin C for prophylaxis of viral hepatitis B in transfused patients. *J. Interntl. Acad. Prev. Med. 5:* 54–58.

Morishige, F., and Murata, A. (1979) Prolongation of survival times in terminal human cancer by administration of supplemental ascorbate. *J. Interntl. Acad. Prev. Med. 5:* 47–52.

Passwater, R. A. (1975) *Supernutrition.* The Dial Press, New York. 224 pages. Advice about nutrition, including the use of nutritional supplements.

Pauling, L. (1968) Orthomolecular psychiatry. *Science 160:* 265–271.

Pauling, L. (1970) Evolution and the need for ascorbic acid. *Proc. Natl. Acad. Sci. USA 67:* 1643–1648.

Pauling, L. (1970) *Vitamin C and the Common Cold.* 122 pages. W. H. Freeman and Co., San Francisco.

Pauling, L. (1976) Vitamin C, the Common Cold, and the Flu. 230 pages. W. H. Freeman and Co., San Francisco.

Pauling, L., et al. (1973) Results of a loading test of ascorbic acid, niacinamide, and pyridoxine in schizophrenic subjects and controls, pages 18–34 in *Orthomolecular Psychiatry: Treatment of Schizophrenia.* Eds: Hawkins, D. and Pauling L. W. H. Freeman and Co., San Francisco.

Pitt, H. A., and Costrini, A. M. (1979) Vitamin C prophylaxis in marine recruits. *J. Am. Med. Assoc. 241:* 988–911.

Priestman, T. J. (1977) Cancer Chemotherapy—An Introduction. Montedison Pharmaceuticals Ltd., Barnet, England.

Rapaport, S. A. (1978) *Strike Back at Cancer: What to Do and Where to Go for the Best Medical Care.* Prentice-Hall, Inc., Englewood Cliffs, New Jersey. 478 pages. Good advice about conventional therapy. No mention of vitamin C.

Rausch, P. G., Pryzwansky, K. B., and Spitznagel, J. K. (1978) Immunocytochemical identification of azurophilic and specific granule markers in the giant granules of Chediak-Higashi neutrophiles. *New Engl. J. Med. 298:* 693–698.

Schlegel, J. U. (1975) Proposed uses of ascorbic acid in prevention of bladder carcinoma. *Ann. N. Y. Acad. Sci. 258:* 432–438.

Schlegel, J. U., Pipkin, G. E., and Banowsky, L. (1967) Urine composition in the etiology of bladder tumor formation. *J. Urol. 97:* 479–481.

Schlegel, J. U., Pipkin, G. E., Nishimura, R., and Duke, G. A. (1969) Studies in the etiology and prevention of bladder carcinoma. J. Urol. *101:* 317–324.

Spero, L. M., and Anderson, T. W. (1973) Ascorbic acid and common colds. *Brit. Med. J. 4:* 354.

Stone, I. (1972) *The Healing Factor: Vitamin C against Disease.* Grosset and Dunlap, New York. 258 pages.

Vallance, S. (1977) Relationships between ascorbic acid and serum proteins of the immune system. *Brit. Med. J. 2:* 437–438.

Watne, A. L., Lai, H-Y, Carrier, J., and Coppula, W. (1977) The diagnosis and surgical treatment of patients with Gardner's syndrome. *Surgery 82:* 327–333.

Weinhouse, S. (1977) Problems in the assessment of human risk of carcinogenesis from chemicals. pp. 1307 to 1309 in *Origins of Human Cancer: Book C, Human Risk Assessment.* Eds: Hiatt, H. H., Watson, J. D. and Winsten, J. A. Cold Spring Harbor Laboratory.

Williams, R. J., and Kalita, D. K., eds. (1977) *A Physician's Handbook on Orthomolecular Medicine.* Pergamon Press, New York. 199 pages. Information about orthomolecular medicine, including advice about vitamin and mineral supplements.

Willis, R. A. (1973) *The Spread of Tumours in the Human Body* (3rd edition). London: Butterworth.

Yonemoto, R. H. (1979) Vitamin C and the immunological response in normal controls and in cancer patients (in Portuguese). *Medico Dialogo 5:* 23–30.

Yonemoto, R. H., Chretien, P. B., and Fehniger, T. F. (1976) Enhanced lymphocyte blastogenesis by oral ascorbic acid. *Proc. Am. Assoc. Cancer Res. 17:* 288.

Name Index

Altman, P. L., 105
Ames, Bruce, 186
Anderson, T. W., 117
Appelbaum, H., 120

Baird, G., xi, 132
Bartlett, M. K., 113
Beatson, George, 71, 73
Becquerel, Henri, 58
Bjelke, E., 187
Breslow, L., 116, 187

Cameron, Ewan, x, xi, xii, xiii, 89, 91,
    117, 129, 132, 133, 140, 142, 152,
    187
Campbell, Allan, xi, xiii, 132, 142, 161
Cartier, Jacques, 99
Cathcart, Robert, 210
Chain, Ernst Boris, 63
Cheraskin, E., 141, 191
Chope, H. D., 116, 187
Chretien, P. B., 110
Cole, Warren H., 56, 93
Coley, William B., 80, 84
Creagan, E. T., 142, 143

DeCosse, J. J., 145
Demole, V., 118
Deucher, W. G., 140
DeVita, Vincent, 134
Dittmer, D. S., 105

Doll, Richard, 184, 188
Domagk, Gerhard, 62
Dvorak, H. F., 110

Ehrlich, Paul, 62
Eijkman, Christiaan, 201
Enstrom, James E., 187
Everson, T. L., 93

Farber, Sidney, 64
Fehniger, T. F., 110
Feigen, George, 109
Fleming, Alexander, 62
Florey, Howard W., 62
Fox, M. S., 55
Funk, Casimir, 201

Gerson, Max, 84, 85, 86, 119
Greer, Edward, 123, 141, 169
Guthy, E. A., 109

Halsted, William, 53, 56
Harris, A., 117
Hopkins, F. Gowland, 201
Horrobin, David, 110
Huggins, Charles, 71, 73

Ivy, Andrew, 84

Jack, T., xiii
Jones, Hardin B., 13, 54, 113

Kalden, J. R., 109
Klenner, Fred R., 100

Lai, H-Y. L., 145
Leibovitz, B., 117
Libby, A. F., xii, 132
Lind, James, 99, 101

McCann, J., 186
McCormick, W. J., 101
McPherson, K., 55
Moertel, Charles G., 133, 142, 194, 195
Morishige, F., 115, 142
Murata, Akira, 115, 142

Pauling, Linus, xii, 89, 91, 112, 114, 117, 133, 140, 187
Pott, Percival, 10

Rapaport, Stephen A., 68
Rausch, P. G., 116
Robinson, Arthur B., 117

Röntgen, Wilhelm Konrad, 58
Rotman, Douglas, x, 129
Ryan, A. E., 113

Schlegel, J. U., 32
Schwerdt, C. E., 115
Schwerdt, P. R., 115
Siegel, B. V., 115
Snow, John, 183
Spero, L., 117
Stone, Irwin, xii, 106, 112, 132, 140
Szent-Györgyi, Albert, 100

Thomas, Lewis, 109

Vallance, S., 109

Watne, A. L., 145
Weinhouse, S., 185
Willis, G. C., 145

Yonemoto, R. H., 110

Subject Index

Actinomycin D, 206
Additives to food, 185, 186, 188
Adenocarcinoma, 19
Adrenal gland, 76
Adrenalectomy, 72
Adrenocorticotropic hormone
(ACTH), 76
Adriamycin, 207
Alcoholic drinks, intake of, 188
Alkeran, 203
Alkylating agents, 67, 203, 204
Amethopterin, 205
Amino acids, 199
Ampoules for vitamin C, 210
Amygdalin, 85, 86
Anaplastic carcinoma, 19
Anaplastic cells, 7
Anastomosis, 191
Angiosarcomas, 39
Animals synthesizing vitamin C, 105
Antibacterial agents, 62
Antibodies, 109
Anticancer drugs, 203–207
Anticoagulant drugs, 110
Antigens, 79
Antimetabolites, 67, 205, 206
Antimitotic antibiotics, 206, 207
Antimitotic vinca alkaloids, 206
Antitoxins, 109
Anus, cancer of, 28
Appendices, 197–214

Appendix carcinoid case history, 150
Appetite, improvement in, xi
Ara-C, 205
Asbestos, 11
Ascorbates. See Vitamin C
Ascorbic acid. See Vitamin C
Aspirin, 102
Astrocytomas, 42
Atrophic gastritis, 23
Autopsy findings, 93
Azaribine, 205

Bacterial vaccines, 81
Basal cell carcinoma, 20
BCG therapy, 81
BCNU, 207
Benign tumor, 18
Beriberi, 201
Beta-naphthylamine, 11
Birth defects, 13
Bladder cancer, 11, 31, 32, 60; case
history of, 173; survival time for,
Fig. 18-3
Blastogenesis, 110
Bleomycin, 207
Blood-forming cells, cancer of, 40–42
Bone pain, 132, 171
Bowels, 119
Brain tumors, 42, 61, 178; case history
of, 170, 171
Breakfast, 188

Breast cancer, 36, 37; case histories of, 149, 160, 162, 163, 171; disseminated, 179; hormones, use of, 70–72; intra-duct carcinoma, 6; minimal response case history, 149; ovaries, removal of, 71; and plasma ascorbate, 124; surgery for, 53–55, 124; survival time for, Fig. 18-2
Bronchus cancer. *See* Lung cancer
Burkitt's lymphoma, 22
Burns from radiotherapy, 192
Busulfan, 204

Carbohydrates, 199
Carcinogenic agents, 10–12
Carcinomas, 19
Carcinosarcomas, 39
Case histories: anecdotal accounts, 168–182; of Vale of Leven patients, 146–167; in U.S. and Canada, 168–182
Causes of cancer, 10–17
CCNU, 207
Cecum carcinoid case history, 150
Cells: anaplastic, 7; causing cancer, 5; chemotherapy affecting, 63, 64; function of, 3, 4; injury, repair after, 4; mutation of, 14; neoplasia, 7; precancer stage, 5, 6; properties of malignancy, 16; structure of, 3; undifferentiated cells showing high mitotic rate, 7
-centesis, defined, 211
Cervical cancer, 60; autopsy findings, 93; pap-smear test, 6
Chediak-Higashi disease, 115
Chemicals: causing cancer, xiii, 12; formula of vitamin C, 208
Chemotherapy, 48, 62–69, 130; and ascorbate treatment, 167, 193–195; and gastrointestinal cancer, 195; and immune system, 142, 143; and plasma ascorbate, 123, 124; and vitamin C, 167, 193–195
Chicken pox, 114
Chlorambucil, 204
Cholera, 183
Cholesterol, 116
Chondroma, 38
Chondrosarcoma, 19, 38
Choriocarcinoma, 42
Chromosomal abnormalities, 15
Chronic leukemias, 41

Cigarette smoke, 11, 12, 31, 185, 187; and heart disease, 116; pancreas, cancer of, 28
Cis-dichlorodimethylplatinum(II), 207
Cis(II)platinum, 207
C_1 esterase, 109
Cobalt 60, 59
Coffee drinkers, 31
Cold sores, 114
Colds and vitamin C, 114
Coley's Fluid, 80, 84
Collagen, 112, 113; fibrils, 129; and radiotherapy, 192
Collagenase, x
Colonic cancer, 25–28; case histories, 153, 154, 159, 160; surgery for, 56; survival time for, Fig. 18-2
Colonic polyposis, 145
Colorectal cancer and 5-FU, 194
Colostomy, 28
Complement complex, 109
Complications of radiation therapy, 60, 61
Complications after surgery, 191
Concentrations of vitamin C, 121
Constitution of patient, 96, 97
Continuous administration of cytotoxic agent, 65, 66
Controlled trials, 133–139
Cortisone, 76, 77
Costs: of cancer, 183; of chemotherapy, 69; of vitamin C, 209
C-Stix, 122
Cure for cancer, 47–49
Cyanocobalamin, 119
Cyclamates, 186
Cyclophosphamide, 204
Cystitis, 191
Cytarabine, 205
Cytosar, 205
Cytosine arabinoside, 205
Cytostasis, case histories of, 152–156
Cytotoxic agents, 64–69
Cytotoxic chemotherapy. *See* Chemotherapy
Cytoxan, 204

DBM, 204
DDP, 207
De novo tumors, 38
Death: from breast cancer, 54, 55; estimate of, 197, 198; statistics on, x

Definition: of medical terms, 18, 19; of surgical terms, 211–216
Depression and vitamin C, 170
DES, 72–74
Detoxifying agent, vitamin C as, 117
Diabetes and *vinca rosea*, 206
Diarrhea, 119, 125
Dibromomannitol, 204
Diet, 199–202; and cancer, 84, 85; and diseases, 201; and gastrointestinal cancer, 187, 195; and laetrile, 85, 86; and plasma ascorbate, 124
DNA molecule, 14
Dosage: most effective, xiii; of vitamin C, 210
Double-blind randomized clinical trial, 133–139
Doxorubicin, 207
Drugs: addictive narcotic, xii; anti-cancer, 203–207; *see also* Chemotherapy
Duodenum, cancer of, 24

-ectomy, defined, 211–212
Embryonal tumors, 43
Emphysema, 186
Encapsulation of tumors, 97, 113
Endometrial cancer, 34
Endoxan, 204
Environmental causes of cancer, 10, 11, 184, 185
Epithelial thickness, precancer stage, 5
Epodyl, 204
Esophagus cancer, 22; and 5-FU, 194
Estrogen, 70–73
Ethoglucid, 204
Evolution and need for Vitamin C, 103–107
Ewing's sarcoma, 38
E-Z Cath, 210

Familial polyposis, 145
Fats, 199
Feedback mechanism, 92
Fermentation, 16
Fever blisters, 114
Fibrin, cocoons of, 110
Fibroid tumor, 38
Fibrosarcoma, 19, 38
Fibrosis, 97
5-Fluorouracil (5-FU), 194, 205
Flatulence, 125
Follicular lymphoma, 39, 40

Food additives, 185, 186
Foods. *See* Diet
Fukuoka Torikai Hospital study, 141, 142

Gallbladder, cancer of, 29; case history, 151
Gastrectomy, 50, 51
Gastrointestinal cancer: and chemotherapy, 195; and diet, 187
Genes, 14; chromosomal abnormalities, 15; point substitution, 14
Gliomas, 42
Glomerular filter, 121
Glossary, 217–222; of surgical terms, 211–216
Glucocorticoids, 76, 77
Glycosaminoglycans, x
-graphy, defined, 212–216
Ground substance, x, 3, 90, 91

Healing process, 4, 112, 113, 191
Heart disease, 116
Heartburn, 125
Heat as cause of cancer, 13, 15
Hematuria, relief from, 132, 173
Hemoglobin-C hemoglobinopathy, 14
Hemorrhage and necrosis of tumor, 163–165
Heparin, 110
Hepatitis, 114, 115
Hepatomegaly, 132
Heredity, 14, 97
High-energy radiation, 59
HN_2, 203
Hodgkin's disease, x, 39, 61; beneficial responses to, 166; case history of, 174; chemotherapy, 68
Homeostasis, 120
Hormone therapy, 70–77, 98, 131; and vitamin C, 192
Host resistance to cancer, 96–98
Hyaluronidase, x, xi, 90, 91, 98, 129; inhibitor of, 92
Hypernephroma, 30
Hypoascorbemia, 106
Hypophysectomy, 72, 74

Immune systems: and chemotherapy, 66, 142, 143, 194; and plasma ascorbate, 124; and surgical dissemination, 190; and vitamin C, 108–111

Immunity, xiii
Immunocompetence, 98
Immunoglobulins, 109
Immunotherapy, 21, 78–82, 193
Induced enzyme formation, 117
Infections after surgery, 191
Infectious diseases and vitamin C, 114, 115
Infiltration, capacity for, 16
Influenza and vitamin C, 114
Intercellular cement, x, 3, 90, 91
Interferon, 114
Intermittent administration of cytotoxic agent, 66
Intestines, 24–28, 170
Intra-cavitary radium therapy, 60
Intravenous fluid, vitamin C in, 113
Intravenous infusion, xiii
Intubation, 23
Invasiveness, 7, 89, 90; controlling, 89–92
Irradiation. See Radiotherapy
Isotopes, use of, 60

Jaundice, 132, 151

Kidney, action of, 121, 122
Kidney adenocarcinomas, 75
Kidney cancer, 30, 31; case history of, 160, 161, 165; surgery, 94; survival time for, Fig. 18-3
Kidney stones, 118
Krebiozen, 84

Laetrile, 85, 86
Larynx, cancer of, 22, 186
L-Asparaginase, 207
Laxative, vitamin C as, 119
Leiomyosarcomas, 38
Leukemia, x, 40–42; acute, 41; case history of, 169, 172; and chemotherapy, 64, 65, 68; hormonal treatment of, 76; misdiagnosis of, 172; radiation therapy, 61
Leukeran, 204
Leukocytes, 110; and Chediak-Higashi disease, 115; and plasma ascorbate, 123, 124
Lip cancer, 60, 186
Lipoma, 39
Lipoprotein cholesterol, 116
Liposarcoma, 19, 39

Liver cancer, 29; and adriamycin, 194, 195
Loading test for ascorbic acid, 122
Lobectomy, 144
Local cancer, 6
Lumpectomy, 54, 55
Lung cancer, 35, 36; in both lungs, 176; case histories, 149–152, 157, 158, 174–176, 181; and cigarette smoking, 11, 12; and radioactive ores, 11; spontaneous regression of, 94; survival time for, Fig. 18-2; Vale of Leven study on, 144
Lymph glands, 7, 8
Lymph nodes, removal of, 53–56
Lymphatic leukemia, 40
Lymphatic system, cancers of, 39, 40
Lymphatics, 7, 8
Lymphocytes, 109, 110; constitutional responses and, 97, 98; hormonal management of, 76
Lymphosarcoma, 39; case history of, 157, 158, 177

Malignant melanoma, 21
Mastectomy, 53–56; and plasma ascorbate, 124
Mayo Clinic trial, 142–144
Measles, 114
Mechlorethamine, 203
Medical x-rays, exposure to, 13
Medulloblastomas, 42
Megavitamin therapy, 103
Melanoma, 21
Melanosarcomas, 39
Melphalan, 203
Meningiomas, 42
Meningitis, 114
Mental state, xi
Merphalan, 203
Mesothelioma, 36; case history of, 178, 179
Metastasis, 8
Methotrexate, 64, 205
MIH, 207
Minerals, 199
Minimal response case histories, 148–150
Mitomycin C, 207
Mitotic inhibitors, 67
Molecular structure and immune system, 108, 109

Moles, malignancy of, 21
MOPP, 67
Mouth cancer, 186
Mule-spinners cancer, 11
Multiple chemotherapy, 67
Multiple myeloma, case history of, 173, 174
Multiple myelomatosis, 41
Multiple portals, radiation through, 59
Mumps, 114
Mustard gas, 64, 203
Mustargen, 203
Mustine, 203
Mutagenicity and carcinogenicity, 186
Mutation of cells, 14
MX, 205
Mycosis fungoides, 173
Myelobromal, 204
Myeloid leukemia, 40; case history of, 169
Myleran, 204
Myoma, 38
Myosarcoma, 19

Narcotic drugs, use of, xii
Narcotics addiction and vitamin C, 132
Nasal sinuses, cancers of, 21
Natulan, 207
Nature of vitamins, 201
Nausea, 125
Necrosis of tumor, 163–166
Neoplasia, 7
Neoplasm, 18, 19
Nephrons, 121
New growth, 18
Night blindness, 201
Nitrates as cause of cancer, 23
Nitrogen mustard, 64, 67, 203
Nitrosamines, 185
Nitrosureas, 207
No response group, 148
Nonmetallic elements, 199
Nutrients, increased amounts of, 17
Nutrition. See Diet
Nutrition therapy, 84, 85

Observer anticipation effect, 83, 131
Occupational cancer, 10, 11
Oligodendrocytomas, 42
-ology, defined, 214, 215
Oncovin, 206
Oophorectomy, 71, 72

Operations. See Surgery
Optimum intake of vitamins, 104, 105–107
Oral contraceptives, 34; gallbladder, cancer of, 29
Orchitis, 114
Organ transplants and immune system, 108
-orrhaphy, defined, 215
Orthomolecular medicine, 70, 102, 103
-oscopy, defined, 215
Osteogenic sarcoma, 19, 37
-ostomy, defined, 215, 216
-otomy, defined, 216
Ovarian cancer, 33; case history of, 146–148, 155, 156; disseminated, 182; hormonal treatment of, 74, 75; and removal of ovaries, 71, 72; survival time for, Fig. 18-3
Over-cautious use of ascorbate treatment, 167
Oxygen, increased amounts of, 16

Pancreas cancer, 28; autopsy findings, 93; case history of, 158, 170
Pap smear, 6, 35, 93
Partial gastrectomy, 50
Penicillin, discovery of, 63
Peritonitis, 191
Periwinkles, 206
Pernicious anemia, 119
-pexy, defined, 216
PGE1, 110
Phagocytic cells, 109, 110
Pharynx, cancers of, 21
Phenylalanine mustard, 203
Pheochromocytoma, 176
PHI, 92
Phosphorus, radioactive isotope of, 60
Physiological hyaluronidase inhibitor, 92
Pigmented mole, malignant, 21
Pipe smoke. See Cigarette smoke
Pituitary gland, removal of, 72
Placebo effect, 83, 131
Plant foods, vitamin content of, 105
Plasma ascorbate, measurement of, 123, 124
-plasty, defined, 216
Pleural effusion: case history of, 176; decrease in, 132

Pleural mesothelioma, case history of, 152

Pneumonia, 115; after surgery, 191; and vitamin C, 114

Poliomyelitis: control of, 184; and vitamin C, 114

Polluted environment and cancer, 184, 185

Polycythermia vera, 41

Polyvinyl chloride (PVC), 29

Precancer stage, 5, 6

Prednisone, 76, 77

Preparation of vitamin C, 208

Prevention of cancer, 17, 183–188

Primary tumor, 6, 7

Procarbazine, 207

Progesterone, 75

Progestogens, 75, 76

Proliferation, capacity for, 16, 89; controlling, 91

Properties of malignancy, 16

Prostaglandin E1, 110

Prostate cancer: autopsy findings, 93; case history of, 157, 158, 171, 172; disseminated, 179, 180; hormonal treatment of, 71, 73, 74

Prostate gland, cancer of, 32, 33

Proteins, 199

Provera, 75

Pulsed-dose technique of chemotherapy, 66

Pumps in kidneys, 121

Purinethol, 205

Radiation as cause of cancer, 13

Radical mastectomy, 53–56

Radioactivity, discovery of, 59

Radiotherapy, 48, 56, 58–61, 131, 140, 141, 191, 192; for lung cancer, 144

Radium needle, implanting of, 60

Raw natural plant foods, vitamin content of, 105

RDAs, 104, 105, 199; Figure II-1, 200

Rebound effect, 117, 118

Recognition of immune system, 108, 109

Recommended dietary allowance of vitamins, 104, 105, 200

Rectum cancer, 25–28; survival time for, Fig. 18-3

Red-cell sedimentation rate, decrease in, 132

References, 223–227

Regression: spontaneous, 9, 21, 93–95, 162; case histories of, 156–163

Remission of leukemia, 172

Research, money for, x

Resistance to cancer, x, 96–98

Retardation of tumor growth case histories, 151, 152

Reticulosis, case history of, 163, 164

Reticulum cell sarcoma, 39; beneficial responses to, 166; case history of, 161, 162

Rhabdomyosarcomas, 38

Rickets, 201

Rodent ulcer, 20

Rupture of surgical wound, 191

Sabin vaccine, 184

Saccharin, 186

Salk vaccine, 184

Sarcomas, 19, 37, 39

Schizophrenia, 122

Scrotal cancer, 10, 11

Scurvy, 99, 100, 201; and cancer, 99–102, 121; and testing for vitamin C, 122, 123

Secondary tumor, 8

Self-prescribed intake of vitamin C, 169, 170

Serratia marcescens, 80

Serum hepatitis, 114, 115

Serum seromucoid level, 132

Shingles, 114

Side effects: of cytotoxic drugs, 66, 68; of DES, 74; of radiotherapy, 191, 192; on spouses of patients, 124; of vitamin C, 118, 119

Signs of cancer, 6

Simple mastectomy, 53, 54, 56

6-Azauridine triacetate, 205

6-Mercaptopurine, 205

6-MP, 205

Skeletal metastases, xii, 132

Skin cancer, 20, 21

Small intestine, cancer of, 24, 25, 180

Smallpox, control of, 183

Smoking, 31, 185, 186

Soft drinks, 188

Solubility of ascorbic acid, 208, 209

Soot as carcinogen, 10

Sources for vitamin C, 209

Spindle-cell sarcoma, 39

Spontaneous regression, 9, 21, 47, 93–95, 162
Spouses of cancer patients and plasma ascorbate, 123–125
Squamous-cell epithelioma, 20
Stage-I cancer, 7
Stage-II cancer, 8
Stage III cancer, 8, 51
Stage IV cancer, 8
Standstill effect. See Cytostasis
Statistics of cancer, x, 10; on lung cancer, 11
Stomach cancer, 23, 24, 50, 51; case histories, 151, 154, 177; and 5-FU, 194; survival time for, Fig. 18-2
Streptococcus cultures, 80
Stress and vitamin C, 120
Sulfur mustard, 203
Sunlight as cause of cancer, 13, 20
Super-radical mastectomy, 53, 54
Surgery, 48, 50–57, 190, 191; complications to, 191; fees charged for, 56; and plasma ascorbate, 124; terms used in, 211–216; value of, 190; and vitamin C, 113
Surgical shock, 113
Surgical terms, 211–216
Survival times, xii, 54; charts of, Fig. 18-2, Fig. 18-3; and number of survivors, Fig. 19-1
Symptoms, 6; of bladder cancer, 3; of colon cancer, 26; of leukemia, 41; of rectum cancer, 27; of stomach cancer, 23
Synoviosarcoma, 19, 38

Table: of controlled trial with cancer patients, Table 18-1; of survival time of terminal patients receiving vitamin C, Table 19-1
Teratomas, 43
Terminal cancer: case histories of, 146–167; treatment of patients with, 129–139
Testicular cancer, 33, 164; hormonal treatment of, 76
Testing for ascorbate status, 122, 123
Thermal agitation, 15
Thiamine, 104
Thioguanine, 206
Thio-Tepa, 204
Throat, cancers of, 21

Thyroid cancer, 60; autopsy findings, 94
Thyroid gland, hormonal treatment of, 75, 76
Thyroxine, 75, 76
Tissue culture, 4
Tissues, effect of radiation on, 58
T-lymphocyte function, 110
Tobacco smoke. See Cigarette smoke
Tongue cancer, 60, 186
Toxic substances, xiii
Transitional-cell papillomatosis, 30
Transplanting organs, 108
Treatment of cancer, 47–49, 189–196
Triethylenethiophosphoramide, 204
TSPA, 204
TTG, 206
Tuberculosis, control of, 183
Tylectomy, 54, 55
Types of cancer, 18

Ultraviolet light, 185; as cause of cancer, 13
Uncontrolled proliferation, 7
Unconventional forms of treatment, 83–86
Undifferentiated cells showing high mitotic rate, 7
Untreatable cancer. See Terminal cancer
Urine: acidity of, 118; and kidneys, 121, 122; loss of vitamin C in, 122; salt in, 120; tested for vitamin C, 122, 123
Uroepithelium, 6
Uterus cancer: cervix, cancer of, 34, 35; endometrial cancer, 34; hormone treatment of, 74, 75

Vaccines against cancer, 184
Vale of Leven Hospital, 129–139; case histories of patients, 146–167; and chemotherapy, 195; lung cancer study, 144
Vascular tumors, beneficial responses to, 166
Velban, 206
Velbe, 206
Vinblastine, 206
Vinca rosea, 206
Vincristine, 206
Viruses, inactivating, xiii
Vitamin A, 81, 188

Vitamin B, 188
Vitamin B1, 104
Vitamin B12, 119
Vitamin C, 81, 99–107; and
    carcinogenic agents, 186; and case
    histories, 146–167; and
    chemotherapy, 193–195; evolution
    and need for, 103–107; and hormone
    therapy, 192; and immune system,
    108–111; and laetrile, 86; optimum
    intake of, 105–107; other properties
    of, 112–119; practical information
    of, 208–210; preparation of, 100;
    and prevention of cancer, 183–188;
    and radiotherapy, 191, 192; side
    effects of, 118–119; and surgery,
    190, 191; and terminal cancer
    patients, 129–139; and treatment of
    cancer, 189–196; in Vale of Leven
    Hospital, 129–139
Vitamin E, 188
Vitamins, defined, 201, 202

Warfarin, 110
Well-being, state of, xi
Well-being of patient, xi, 131
Wound healing and vitamin C, 112,
    113, 191

X-rays: chromosomal abnormalities,
    15; discovery of, 58; exposure to, 13;
    radiotherapy, see Radiotherapy

**Here are two books every
health-conscious person should have:**

EARL MINDELL'S
VITAMIN BIBLE

SUGAR BLUES

Earl Mindell, a certified nutritionist and practicing pharmacist for over fifteen years, heads his own national company specializing in vitamins. His VITAMIN BIBLE is the most comprehensive and complete book about vitamins and nutrient supplements ever written. This important book will reveal:

- How vitamin needs vary for each of us and how to determine yours

- What special food cravings can mean about your vitamin needs

- How to substitute natural substances for tranquilizers, sleeping pills and other drugs

- How the right vitamins can help your heart

- How vitamins can retard aging

- How vitamins and nutrient supplements can improve sex

Do you know that sugar is an addictive, destructive drug like opium, morphine and heroin, yet Americans consume it daily in everything from cigarettes to bread. William Dufty, once a sugar addict himself, has, under Gloria Swanson's influence, kicked the sugar habit. He tells you how, if you are overweight or suffer from migraine, hypoglycemia or acne, the Sugar Blues have hit you.... and how you too can kick the habit. This eye-opening book shows you how to live better without the insidious poison of sugar and includes recipes for delicious dishes—all sugar-free.

Available in paperback
　　　　L93613-8　$2.95

Available in paperback
　　　　L93786-X　$2.95

A doctor tells you the truth about doctors and medicine in:

CONFESSIONS OF A MEDICAL HERETIC

Dr. Robert S. Mendelsohn is Chairman of the Medical Licensing Committee for the State of Illinois, Associate Professor of Preventive Medicine and Community Health in the School of Medicine of the University of Illinois and the recipient of numerous awards for excellence in medicine and medical instruction. And Dr. Mendelsohn tells you how to make your own decision regarding your medical treatment.

Dr. Mendelsohn explains why he is convinced that:

- Annual physical examinations are a health risk
- Hospitals are dangerous places for the sick
- Most operations do little good and many do harm
- Medical testing laboratories are scandalously inaccurate
- Many drugs cause more problems than they cure
- The X-ray machine is the most pervasive and most dangerous tool in the doctor's office

It is *your* health that is at stake!

Available in paperback   L95554-2 $2.75